# THE
# PSYCHIATRIST
# IN COURT

## A Survival Guide

# THE PSYCHIATRIST IN COURT

## A Survival Guide

**Thomas G. Gutheil, M.D.**
Harvard Medical School
Boston, Massachusetts

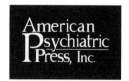

Washington, DC
London, England

**Note:** The authors have worked to ensure that all information in this book concerning drug dosages, schedules, and routes of administration is accurate as of the time of publication and consistent with standards set by the U.S. Food and Drug Administration and the general medical community. As medical research and practice advance, however, therapeutic standards may change. For this reason and because human and mechanical errors sometimes occur, we recommend that readers follow the advice of a physician who is directly involved in their care or the care of a member of their family.

Books published by the American Psychiatric Press, Inc., represent the views and opinions of the individual authors and do not necessarily represent the policies and opinions of the Press or the American Psychiatric Association.

Copyright © 1998 American Psychiatric Press, Inc.
ALL RIGHTS RESERVED
Manufactured in the United States of America on acid-free paper
First Edition
01   00   99   98      4   3   2

American Psychiatric Press, Inc.
1400 K Street, N.W., Washington, DC   20005
www.appi.org

**Library of Congress Cataloging-in-Publication Data**
Gutheil, Thomas G.
     The psychiatrist in court : a survival guide / Thomas G. Gutheil.
         p.      cm.
     Includes bibliographical references and index.
     ISBN 0-88048-764-X (alk. paper)
     1. Forensic psychiatry—United States—Popular works.
     2. Evidence, Expert—United States—Popular works.   I. Title.
     [DNLM: W 740 G984pa 1998]
KF8965.Z9G88   1998
347.73′67—dc21
DNLM/DLC
for Library of Congress                                           97-34483
                                                                              CIP

**British Library Cataloguing in Publication Data**
A CIP record is available from the British Library.
Cover image copyright © 1997 PhotoDisc, Inc.

# About the Author

Thomas G. Gutheil, M.D., is Professor of Psychiatry at Harvard Medical School, Codirector of the Program in Psychiatry and the Law at the Massachusetts Mental Health Center, and a Fellow of the American Psychiatric Association. He is the first Professor of Psychiatry in the history of Harvard Medical School to be board certified in both general and forensic psychiatry. Through more than 200 publications and international lectures and seminars, he has taught many clinicians about the interfaces between psychiatry and the law. He has received local and national teaching awards, and his textbook *Clinical Handbook of Psychiatry and the Law*, co-authored with Paul S. Appelbaum, M.D., received the Manfred S. Guttmacher Award as the outstanding contribution to forensic psychiatric literature.

*To my family,*
*for putting up with*
*this labor and vocation.*

# Contents

# 4
—

# 5
—

# 6
---

# 7
---

# 8

## Specific Roles for the Psychiatrist in Court . . . . . 77

# 9

## Epilogue . . . . . . . . . . . . . . . . . . . . 91

# APPENDIX 1

## On Wearing Two Hats: Role Conflict in Serving as Both Psychotherapist and Expert Witness . . . . . . 93

*Larry H. Strasburger, M.D., Thomas G. Gutheil, M.D.
and Archie Brodsky, B.A.*

# APPENDIX 2

# Acknowledgments

I am indebted to members of the Program in Psychiatry and the Law, Massachusetts Mental Health Center, for years of stimulating dialogues that formed the substrate for this work and especially to Drs. Steven Behnke, Douglas Ingram, Larry Strasburger, and Shannon Woolley for their meticulous reading of the manuscript and their detailed, thoughtful, and supremely helpful critical suggestions and comments. My deep thanks to Ms. Ellen Lewy for her skilled and patient assistance with this manuscript.

# 1

# Introduction: "What? Me? Go to Court?"

For the practicing psychiatrist, the prospect of going to court under any circumstances at any time for any reason is as welcome an idea as dentistry without anesthesia. Huddled around lunchroom tables in the hospital cafeteria, trembling physicians share lurid tales of colleagues dragged into court by some subterfuge and then, metaphorically, drawn asunder by teams of wild Caucasian horses on the witness stand at the merciless orchestration of—the attorney.

But the facts are inescapable: citizens are flocking to court in ever-increasing numbers for an ever-expanding set of reasons.

Some of those would-be litigants are our patients, who may even—Heaven forbid—sue us in malpractice cases. Even without such an outcome, however, ordinary psychiatrists working in the trenches of patient care may be swept into the courtroom in some other rush to judgment, such as your patient suing someone else or a custody struggle ensuing when marital counseling fails. If you are one of those so swept, I am confident you would agree that some guidance would be useful.

This book surely will not turn any psychiatrist into someone who loves to go to court—that goal is probably beyond the power of any book—but it may decrease the terror. Knowledge is not only power but also an antidote to unreasoning fear. Hence, my purpose is to help you, the psychiatrist-reader, become more knowledgeable about the setting, the assumptions, the personnel, and the issues and techniques involved in going to court, with the aim of demystifying and reducing your anxiety about this stressful experience.

Practically, this book is aimed at the practitioner whose knowledge about going to court is limited to television and movies. At times my review may seem a bit basic, but I find in teaching audiences of our peers and colleagues that it is best to start from the most rudimentary position. Not only does that approach include everyone in the audience, but it also may correct misperceptions and distortions introduced by the media. Hollywood, after all, is not reality as we know it.

Beginning with some introductory information about the basics of the legal process and its personnel, I then discuss some threshold issues such as the subpoena; I describe the different types of witnesses, how to work with your attorney, and how to write reports for the courtroom. The final topics in this book are actual approaches to testifying on the witness stand and a discussion of a number of roles that a psychiatrist may play in court procedure. In these discussions, I have attempted to achieve as much verisimilitude as possible by drawing examples directly from hundreds of actual cases and countless consultations with peers and colleagues on how to deal with the legal system.

Finally, three principles have shaped the form of this book.

First, it is written in an informal, demystifying, and even light-hearted tone for easier mental access and for a soothing, supportive effect intentionally designed to allay your anxiety. Second, the focus is constantly on the practical rather than theoretical issues. Third, the book is short enough so that you could read it all, if pressed, between the arrival of the subpoena and the court appearance.

I hope that—although nothing can make participation in the legal process pleasant—reading this book may make going to court less traumatic, perhaps even something of an adventure. Good luck on your next time in court.

# 2

# The Courtroom as Foreign Country

**P**retend for a moment that your normally restful sleep is interrupted by a most disturbing dream. You find yourself standing on a high elevation in front of a crowd of people who are staring at you, perhaps because you are stark naked. People bark what appear to be questions at you about something that seems to be of great importance and meaning, but they are speaking a strange language so that you cannot determine what is going on and are thus helpless to respond.

To the clinician whose native turf is the quiet, familiar private practice office, the courtroom, like few other places on earth,

---

The author acknowledges valuable input to this chapter by James T. Hilliard, Esq., leading health care attorney.

presents the classic feelings of strangeness, helplessness, and nakedness typical of the worst nightmare. Being on the witness stand combines all the primal fears: being exposed, being helpless, speaking in public, not knowing the rules or the ropes, being made to look foolish, being intimidated, and so on.

To help you with these fears, let me propose a model for your first venture into court: treat it as though you were an American going to a mildly hostile, mildly intolerant, chauvinistic foreign country where they dress and speak quite differently—for example, France. Your basic survival strategies would probably include studying important customs before your trip; becoming somewhat familiar with the language, especially some key phrases ("Pardonnez-moi, s'il vous plaît, ou est le WC?"); getting acquainted with cultural assumptions and taboos; and perhaps educating yourself on the proper dress code for various situations. Although such anticipatory approaches would not solve all your problems, they would be likely to reduce them to manageable proportions. Such survival strategies also may make appearing in the foreign land of court less stressful; indeed, that is the very purpose of this book.

In this chapter, I discuss some of the basic cultural assumptions of the foreign country that is court, with the goal of decreasing the strangeness of it all and of lowering your anxiety about traveling there.

## Fun With Your Tame Attorney

In foreign countries you may not know which parts of the city are safe or which lovely forest glade may turn out to be quicksand. Surely a guide would be helpful; in the legal system, we call such guides attorneys. One of the most reassuring and supportive factors in dealing with the foreign country that is the legal system is the assistance of a capable attorney as a native guide. Your attorney can be of enormous assistance in helping you find your way and understanding the strange linguistic turns given even to your own language. In today's litigious society, every clinician should have access to an attorney experienced in mental health law or at least in common psychiatric legal issues.

The title of this discussion is meant to indicate that clinicians will have the best handle on problematic situations that may arise at the medicolegal interface by developing a cordial relationship with the attorney on a regular basis well in advance of urgent need (hence, "tame attorney"). It is well worth your time and effort to canvass your professional colleagues for those attorneys who are the solid citizens in this field and to spend a lunch or two meeting and discussing with such an attorney your career goals, type of practice, and so on. Mutual referrals may ensue; inviting the attorney to address your professional society or practice group on a subject of current interest is an excellent icebreaker and a way to offer potential business contacts to the attorney.

The purpose of all this socializing is to move the attorney into the acquaintance category so that when disaster strikes and you have to call on someone, he or she will not be a stranger.

If a medicolegal question arises before you have a chance to cultivate such a relationship, consider calling your malpractice insurance company and asking to talk to one of its favorite law firms. Because insurance companies (may I speak frankly here?) are not in business to lose money, the attorneys from the company's customary law firms are not graduates just out of law school but practitioners highly experienced and thoroughly versed in medicolegal matters.

Legal consultation services exist in connection with insurers, the American Psychiatric Association, and other groups. Although not the same as an attorney who is a personal acquaintance, such resources can be valuable, particularly to practitioners who practice in high-risk situations.

Finally, if you will forgive a personal bias, don't forget the value of consultation with a forensic psychiatrist or a psychiatrist versed in medicolegal issues. The chances are greater that the advice you are given will rest on a firm *clinical* foundation—a definite advantage.

Having said all that, I note that attorneys also can bring one to grief, especially through failure to check out sources from the beginning. An unsuspecting clinician may receive a call from a person identifying himself or herself as "the attorney on the (patient's name) case"; only later, after having conversed freely with the attorney, does the clinician learn that the attorney was on the *opposing* side of the patient's case, and significant inappropriate disclosure or other harm may have been done. Be alert to such fishing expeditions, which may not be seen as unethical by attorneys.

In this regard, if an attorney contacts you, request that he or she identify the client. If you have the slightest doubt about who the client is or what the client's interests are in the case, call your own attorney before any further disclosures.

Recall that even the patient's own attorney is not routinely or automatically entitled to clinical information about the patient without explicit, preferably written, permission.

## A Personal Attorney?

Let us say that you are not consulting the attorney because your patient is involved in some legal matter but because you are actually being sued by one of your patients. A question that frequently arises in this situation is whether you need a personal attorney over and above the one supplied by the malpractice insurance carrier if you are being sued in a malpractice action. The short answer is no if you are a full-time private practitioner; maybe, if you are a clinician who works in an institution or agency. The latter case depends on whether the interests of the agency (hospital or clinic, for example) might diverge from your own interests. Because this could theoretically occur at any point, one rule of thumb is if the carrier supplies one lawyer for two defendants—you and the hospital or clinic—it is usually wise to have your own lawyer.

Two other aspects of this matter merit comment here. Having your own lawyer already does not mean that he or she will be defending you in the case. The insurer decides, for the most part, who the attorney will be. Engaging your own lawyer would be primarily for personal consultation and reality testing throughout the legal process. Indeed, not all attorneys assigned to defend malpractice cases are able or willing to deal with the anxieties experienced during your first-ever malpractice case. In certain instances, therefore, you may wish to engage your own attorney for consulting purposes and anxiety control. The best native guide, after all, not only directs but also supports and encourages the traveler in the foreign country.

You must, however, be sure to notify the insurance carrier for the agency early on. If you work for a state or federal agency or institution, you may enjoy the protection of tort claims acts, which often contain provisions (caps on awards, immunities, or other limits on litigation). However, if your own private attorney independently takes some legal actions that the agency's insurer views as prejudicing its defense of your case, you may be "cut loose" as a defendant under the agency and therefore may be unprotected by the umbrella of protections that you might otherwise have enjoyed because of your position in the agency. Clearly, legal consultation at a minimum is essential to your protection.

In any case, regardless of your consulting with or engaging your own attorney upon learning you are about to be sued, it is imperative that —by following your private attorney's advice—you do not prejudice your contractual relationship with your malpractice insurer or if you work for a state, local, or federal government, with the tort claims process. Clear your actions with both sets of attorneys. Early notification and cooperation with your insurer are crucial. Your private attorney should do nothing absent an emergency (for example, to meet filing deadlines) that would interfere with or give your insurance carrier cause to deny coverage.

## Some Notes on Malpractice

Psychiatrists have always enjoyed a place low on the list of medical specialties being sued for malpractice, but *low* is not *none*. Historically, suicide cases—wherein a patient has committed (or even attempted) suicide and the family brings suit against the practitioner—have been the leading claim against mental health professionals of all disciplines. That primacy still exists.

Sexual misconduct cases and, lately, cases alleging harm from boundary violations without actual intercourse are on the rise as the second or third most common claim; more precisely, complaints for *sexual* boundary violations are down, although those for *nonsexual* boundary violations are up, according to the American Psychiatric Association Ethics Committee. Cases for breach of confidentiality, misdiagnosis and mistreatment (especially pharmacology and "recovered memory"), and harm to third parties are among the more frequently occurring claims, but the order changes every year.

Managed care has raised an entire class of cases into new prominence by some mechanism such as the following: an ordinary suicide case or negligent treatment case is complicated by the *time* allowed for hospitalization or treatment of the patient. For example, if a patient is discharged at the expiration of coverage and later commits suicide, the claim can be advanced that—had the insurance been greater or the practitioner willing to continue treatment—more treatment should have been undertaken, a longer stay might have been possible, and the suicide might not have occurred. This kind of case adds a financial dimension to treatment that sets a disturbing tone for modern juries, who traditionally refuse to hear about limits on care.

Such cases are so much on the upswing that a well-known mental health law attorney has given up all other areas of practice and now makes a good living solely on cases of disgruntled managed care customers suing the agencies or the providers.

A more detailed exploration of current malpractice issues is beyond the scope of this book; suffice it to say that litigation is alive and well and may well be the reason for which you, the reader, find use for this text.

# 3

## Personnel and Procedures of the Courtroom

$\mathbf{A}$lthough the "players" may vary somewhat, depending on the type of legal function being accomplished, some basic roles remain the same.

First, there is the linchpin of the proceedings: a decision maker, called the **fact finder.** The fact finder may be a judge alone in a civil or criminal case, a judge plus a jury, or—in some proceedings, such as a case before a medical licensing board in some states—an administrative law judge.

Recall that a criminal trial is about the moral blameworthiness of someone who has broken the law or violated a statute. In contrast, civil litigation is not about blameworthiness (although defendants in malpractice suits will immediately note that it sure feels as though it were); instead, civil litigation is about compensating for losses, harms, or wrongs. The law refers to this compensation as making someone "whole"; if A loses a leg through B's negligence, for example, the money accruing from the civil suit is supposed to compensate for the lost leg and make A whole again.

All the varieties of judge previously listed are addressed as "Judge," "Judge Jones," or, mostly, "Your Honor" and are thanked regularly; indeed, the proper response to most remarks that the judge may address to you is "Thank you, Your Honor," with few exceptions:

> *Judge:* Doctor, now that you have been sworn in, counsel will ask you some questions.
> *You:* Thank you, Your Honor.
> *Judge:* Also, please try to keep your voice up as the acoustics in this room are pretty bad.
> *You:* Thank you, Your Honor.
> *Judge:* Now then, please state your name for the record.
> *You (carried away):* Thank you, Your Honor.

One of the "foreign" aspects of the judge's role is the sometimes confusing tendency to be identified in the second or third person in courtroom parlance. For example, if an attorney is asking for some special consideration from the judge, he or she does not say, "If you would be so kind, . . . " Instead, that request is, "If Your Honor please" or "May it please the court." The judge, too, uses the third person referring to himself or herself, as in "The court finds that that evidence is inadmissible" rather than "*I* find. . . . "

Next are the **attorneys,** of which there are almost always two or two sets, because we have in the United States an adversarial system (see "Some Basic Rules" later in this chapter). These are addressed as "Counselor" or "Mr. Smith" or "Ms. Jones" and are thanked, if at all, only when they do you some favor, such as refilling your water glass.

The novice witness may be confused by multiple attorneys, who are a common feature of malpractice suits. Let us say a patient is suing a therapist-counselor, a social worker, and a medical backup physician, all of whom practice at a hospital. The therapist, the social worker, the physician, and the hospital may each be represented by different attorneys under the theory that the interests of these parties may well be separate and may diverge, even though it is common practice for attorneys for an associated group of treaters to hang together.

Don't be thrown by the occasional archaism of an attorney's referring to another attorney as "my brother" or "my sister." This reference doesn't convey relatedness by blood; it is merely a traditional variant on "my colleague."

Commonly, but not always, a **clerk** of the court is located near the judge. The clerk has a variety of functions, ranging from judge's gofer to legal researcher; most often he or she takes notes, hands the judge relevant documents, checks that witnesses are present, takes telephone calls for the judge, and marks exhibits (that is, identifies with colored and numbered tags those documents or pieces of physical evidence that will be formally included and admitted as evidence in this proceeding).

A **bailiff** also may be present, sometimes in a police officer–, sheriff–, or security guard–like uniform; his or her job is to keep order and prevent disgruntled witnesses, plaintiffs, or defendants from attacking anyone in court. The bailiff commonly announces that court is in session and may announce the arrival of judge or jury.

A **stenographer** is usually present with a stenotype machine or some other form of recording apparatus (such as a tape recorder) to preserve a record of the proceedings. It is a much-appreciated courtesy for the psychiatrist-witness to spell technical words and unusual names for the stenographer's benefit; this advice stands in addition to the basic rule: speak slowly and clearly. Some additional tips on this topic are discussed in Chapter 5 in this volume.

The oath sworn by the witness to tell the truth may be administered by the clerk, the stenographer, the judge, or, more rarely, the bailiff. The seriousness of this step—that is, the penalty of perjury for false statements under oath—is the same regardless.

Recent authors of sociological studies on lying have reported its universality in human affairs, but the common conversational lie is a matter of personal moral outlook. The critical importance of truth telling in legal matters, however, alters profoundly the moral and legal context. *Perjury* is defined in the present context as lying in court while under oath. It is a serious crime that may itself be the subject of a trial, with serious penalties for a finding of guilt.

The **jury** is historically intended to represent a "biopsy" of the community, which votes its conscience in the proceeding. Although there are exceptions to the rule, a jury often is composed of individuals of approximately a ninth-grade level education. In some communities, there may be occasions when all members of the jury are college graduates, but these occasions should be considered rare. This empirical fact places some weight on the witness's paying attention to language level and vocabulary, as will be examined later in this chapter.

Under ideal circumstances, the judge is a former senior and skilled attorney chosen, appointed, or, in some areas, elected because of superior intelligence and wisdom, exceptional knowledge of the law, incorruptible fairness, and objectivity. In other jurisdictions, the judge may be, as one Boston attorney put it, "a lawyer whose brother-in-law is the governor." Regardless, the judge rules the courtroom. Whatever failings or foibles the judge may reveal—I once had the terrifying experience of a judge undergoing a paranoid decompensation while asking me some questions directly—the court carries on. Serious errors must wait to be remedied at the appeals-court level.

Finally, there are the **parties,** the central players in the case. In civil cases, the parties are the **plaintiff(s)** and the **defendant(s).** In criminal trials, the accused person is the defendant; the prosecution may be the federal government, the state, the city, or the county; and the attorney may be the attorney general or district attorney. In administrative proceedings (for example, against a physician's license), the parties may be the physician and the board of licensure, each represented by an attorney. In an ethics complaint, the physician and the ethics committee of the relevant professional organization itself may or may not retain attorneys.

One final person seen less often is the **guardian ad litem,** or GAL. The word *litem* is etymologically related to *litigation.* The GAL is usually an attorney (but may be a physician or psychiatrist under some circumstances) who has a wide range of functions intended to aid the court in gathering information. These functions may include investigating a situation for the court as to whether a certain person, place, or situation actually exists where it is supposed to be (for example, is there such a person at a particular nursing home, and does he or she really need a guardian as claimed?); opposing the moving party in a proceeding to provide balance to the issue (such as challenging involuntary medication of an inpatient); or filling in to represent the interests of any party who otherwise would not have legal representation (for example, representing a fetus in an abortion case). Because of direct judicial appointment in some cases, the GAL may be outside the immediate adversary framework; from the witness's viewpoint, GALs generally should be treated as if they were attorneys in the case until told otherwise.

## Some Basic Rules

Like any social system, the courtroom has a set of basic rules and assumptions that are not always explained in detail. A working familiarity with these fundamentals will aid considerably in increasing the confidence of the novice witness.

The fundamental principle, if there is one, is the notion of the adversary system or model. This is the basic axiom that the path to legal truth is obtained by having the two sides of the cases in question draw apart the evidence—literally.

To grasp more clearly what the practical impact of this model may be, consider treatment planning in the clinical inpatient setting. If the treatment team consists of five members, experience shows that there will probably be five views of the patient and five opinions as to how that patient can best be treated. The team leader or the team as a whole, however, must reach a consensus so that coherent treatment can proceed. The wrangling of the penta-logue, as it were (that is, fight among the team members), must result in a best solution, even if it is a compromise. In the court-room, the two sides battle in a zero-sum game—one winner, one loser—and only one party's interests prevail.

Another implication of this model is the way in which ambiva-lence is treated. In real life, a given person may be ambivalent about a wish, even a wish for compensation. In court, no such am-bivalence is expressed—you sue only to win. Arguments opposing your wish belong to the "other side." These arguments can lead to some stresses for the psychiatrist testifying about a patient's men-tal state, with all the complexity, ambivalence, and multiply-driven nature of the human condition. Such complexities do not fit easily into the Procrustean confines of the adversary model.

A second basic assumption that consultative experience shows to be problematic for the novice witness is the idea of the selective admissibility of evidence. In clinical planning, again, all input is desirable although it may be accorded different weight. The views, observations, and interview data of even the most junior member of the team (for example, the medical student) are sought and welcomed as part of the totality of clinical input to decision mak-ing. Half-recalled memories—of what the patient's second cousin may have said, as reported by the mother to the social work stu-dent and then passed on to the social worker who shares it with the team—may constitute valuable clinical data, despite the con-voluted, hearsay-ridden trail by which it comes to the team's attention.

In contrast, an important component of the perceived essential fairness of the legal system is the mechanism by which evidence makes it into court. Fairness is seen to demand exclusion of even some concrete evidence in the name of justice. Experience reveals that this exclusion is a particularly frustrating aspect of the pro-ceedings for clinicians going into court. Despite taking an oath to tell "the whole truth," and despite the clinician's wish that the en-tire story of his or her patient be told to the court for full under-standing, the extent of the information to which the witness can testify may be severely circumscribed:

A clinician was testifying in court for the second time about a case; the previous case had ended in a mistrial. To reveal this fact, however, would have been deemed prejudicial to the jury. As a result, complex locutions such as "in previous sworn testimony" had to be agreed on to refer to the earlier trial.

The need to adapt one's narrative impulses to the requirements of the legal system can place great strain on novice witnesses, especially those whose emotions have already been inflamed by the strangeness of the courtroom, the system's often callous treatment of the mentally ill , and the occasionally abusive nature of interrogation by attorneys. Passionate feelings, however, do not justify attempting to force the court to hear what one believes it should. The rule in the legal system is to answer all the questions, then sit down. Judges are notoriously intolerant of anything that smacks of disruption or of preempting their authority, and the psychiatrist who demands to be heard risks citation for contempt of court.

This last issue alerts us to another core assumption of the courtroom: its Socratic aspect. Although there are many possible ways of telling a story, discussing a conflictful subject, or reaching the truth, the legal method is that of question and answer (note as a curiosity that the Anglo-Saxon etymology of the word *answer* is "swear to"). It may be useful to contrast this model with the one more familiar to the clinician: the case presentation or write-up. The organization of the latter follows a narrative flow organized into sections, which are essentially extended paragraphs: chief complaint, history of the present illness, psychiatric history, family history, and so on. A hypothetical case presentation in the clinical context might be

The patient, John Smith, is a 35-year-old white Protestant male who came to treatment with me on October 15, 1991, for depression and anxiety. I started him on a regimen of Prozac and psychotherapy, and he responded well. . . .

Although there is occasionally room for narratives like that in the courtroom setting, this crisp monologue might well be replaced by an equally crisp but more extensive dialogue, governed by considerations that go beyond simply getting the facts out there. For example, the questions asked cannot be leading, on the one hand (a question is deemed "leading" when the actual or expected answer is contained within the question, as in "You gave him 50 mg of Thorazine, did you not?"); on the other hand, questions may be used to define legally relevant points. The questions should not appear to make assumptions that have not yet been established, which leads to some strange-sounding locutions. Consider the following:

> *Attorney:* Doctor, are you familiar with an individual named John Smith? (The attorney, and sometimes the entire courtroom, may already know this, because Smith may have already testified to this effect and the point may not be contested; it doesn't matter. This question is part of a background-supplying procedure known as "laying a foundation," on top of which future factual structures may be built.)
>
> *Physician-witness:* Yes.
>
> *Attorney:* Can you point him out to us?
>
> *Physician-witness:* There (points).
>
> *Attorney:* Let the record reflect that Dr. Jones has pointed to the plaintiff. (This locution, of course, deals with the fact that the physician's index finger is not visible on the written transcript.) Now Doctor, when did you first encounter Mr. Smith?
>
> *Physician-witness:* October 15, 1991.
>
> *Attorney:* And how did that come about? (This question is another redundancy, undisputed, already established—but not with this witness.)
>
> *Physician-witness:* He came in for a consultation.
>
> *Attorney:* And where did that take place? (Again, it probably did not take place in a telephone booth, but each element of the facts needs to be clearly established.)
>
> *Physician-witness:* In my office at Mercy Hospital.

*Attorney:* When Mr. Smith came to consult you on October 15, 1991, what, if anything, did he tell you he had come for? (Although it is unlikely that Mr. Smith came for the consultation and said nothing—although that does happen in psychiatry—the phrasing is couched so as not to make the assumption that something was said. Note also that queries such as "Why did he come to see you?" or "What did he come for?" are less proper because they leave unarticulated for the record how the physician would know. Reciprocally, the witness's answer also should address this point.)

*Physician-witness:* He told me that he had been depressed for a number of weeks and that he was troubled by anxiety (rather than "depression and anxiety"; the physician, also, avoids appearing to know or to assume any ultimate truth beyond what the patient said).

*Attorney:* And did you, in fact, undertake a consultation?

*Physician-witness:* Yes, I did. (This last exchange, although perhaps logical and even redundant, is doubly necessary. First, the form of the question doesn't assume that a consultation automatically took place; maybe, somehow, it didn't. But more significantly and less obviously, the phrase "did you, in fact, undertake a consultation" in this context represents an offer of care such as might establish a physician-patient relationship and the accompanying duty, relevant in a malpractice context, to render nonnegligent care.)

*Attorney:* And what, if any, treatment did you administer? (The "if any" may sound to the novice witness like sarcasm or even like an implication that this physician would not treat a sick person who came for help; it is neither. Again, this phrasing avoids creating the assumption by means of the question that treatment was, in fact, administered.)

> *Physician-witness:* I started him on Prozac and psycho-
>    therapy.
> *Attorney:* And how long was Mr. Smith treating with
>    you? (For reasons that remain totally unexplained,
>    this awkward-sounding locution, "treating with,"
>    appears universally used by attorneys questioning
>    treating psychiatrists.)

In later queries, the physician would be asked to define and explain both treatment modalities, to address the effects, and so on.
Although it might be arguably faster to let the physician just spit
out the story (and this is occasionally done with some expert witnesses), the central method of obtaining testimony and building
brick by brick the edifice of evidence remains the question and
answer.

## Subpoenas, Privilege, and
## Other Threshold Questions

Clinicians list as one of the scariest experiences in their careers the
receipt of a subpoena in the mail or by hand from a constable or
other official. Much of this fear appears based on what the subpoena is not (that is, an arrest). Because the subpoena represents
one of many pathways to the courtroom, I review it in this chapter.
    Subpoenas are of two varieties: the regular subpoena and the
subpoena duces tecum. The word *subpoena* means "under penalty"; the concept is that you must appear in court under penalty
of the law, for example, by being held in contempt of court. The
phrase *duces tecum* from the Latin ("may you bring with you")
means that when you appear, you must bring with you to court
some relevant material, such as a patient's record or correspon-
dence. You may receive a fully expected subpoena for a carefully
prearranged court appearance as a kind of formality, or one may
descend on you from out of the blue.
    On the one hand, the subpoena is no big deal; attorneys have

them on standard pads like prescription blanks and issue them as needed. However, you cannot ignore a subpoena; you must respond in some way, but the way you respond may not necessarily mean going to court. Your attorney's guidance will be particularly helpful here.

On receiving a subpoena unexpectedly, first call the clerk of the court from which the subpoena has been issued and ask what it is about. The reason for this inquiry is that it may be impossible to tell from the jumble of jargon on the papers themselves just what the whole matter concerns. For example, you may know of a patient who died while under your care, but you may not recognize on the subpoena the name of the executor of the patient's estate, nor connect it with the name of the patient on whose behalf your presence in court is being solicited.

Under various circumstances, you may wish (or you may be advised by your attorney) to cancel the subpoena legally; this action is called *quashing* the subpoena, the legal counter maneuver to the subpoena itself. Under other circumstances, your patient's attorney, the patient's spouse's attorney, or some other figure may attempt to quash the subpoena. It is also possible to negotiate with the clerk for a less disruptive, more convenient, and more planned court appearance time than the one initially prescribed on the document.

In considering the subpoena duces tecum, whereby material must be brought into the courtroom, keep in mind that the subpoena merely gets some form of evidence into the courtroom; after that point, other considerations may apply. For example, the clinician who is asked by means of a subpoena duces tecum to bring a patient's medical record to court should not then immediately thrust the record into the first outstretched hand he or she encounters. Constraints may exist within the system to prevent release at all, or release to or beyond a certain extent, of the materials. To grasp this issue, consider briefly the concept of privilege.

Privilege is often contrasted with confidentiality. The latter represents an ethical obligation of the clinician to keep matters revealed during clinical work in confidence (that is, from third parties), absent permission to reveal it. In contrast, *privilege* is a right belonging to patients (in the present context) whereby they may bar material shared with clinicians from emerging in legal or quasi-legal settings. That is, a patient exerts or exercises a privilege to keep things out of the courtroom (or its equivalents, such as hearings and depositions).

The laws pertaining to privilege are complex and riddled with exceptions, such that most nonattorneys cannot be expected to know about them. As a result, as a practical matter, privilege decisions are usually a contest between attorneys, resolved by the judge, as in the following example:

> A husband and wife were engaged in a custody fight. During the divorce proceedings, the husband had sought psychiatric treatment to deal with the stresses of the dissolving marriage. The wife attempted to subpoena the husband's treatment records in the hopes of using the material to cast aspersions on his fitness for parenting. The husband tried to assert a therapist-patient privilege (available in some jurisdictions) to keep the records out of court. The judge ruled that he would review the records *in camera* (that is, in private chambers off the record rather than in open court) to determine their relevance. The judge ultimately ruled that the records were not relevant, so they were, in fact, excluded.

Beyond the matter of privilege, other forces may affect the admissibility of clinical data. In some jurisdictions, for example, a court order rather than a subpoena is required to produce a medical record, especially against the wishes of the patient in question. These issues are problems for the attorney and are not reviewed in this chapter. One caution applies to both presentation of courtroom data and record keeping itself: the importance of distinguishing among sources of clinical data. In practice, this means both being clear in your mind and recording clearly in your notes where certain information comes from. Important distinctions, for example, apply to data reported secondhand ("My mother said to me . . . "), thirdhand ("The nurse reported that the patient said . . . "), and direct observation ("The patient appeared for her appointment pale and tremulous . . . ").

A distinction must even be made between clinical and legal

"facts." You intuitively know what a fact is, at least until you have to explain it in court. What makes this matter even more complicated is that the legal system uses the term *fact* to refer not only to the points (factual elements) on which the decision maker bases his or her conclusion but also to the conclusion itself. Such use of this term is why the judge, for instance, is referred to as a fact finder when that term really means decision maker, outcome determiner, or conclusion generator, which can lead to confusing dialogues.

For example, in a custody battle in which child sexual abuse was claimed, the expert witness testified about how elements of the case were consistent, according to a forensic analysis, with the claim being false or unfounded. The judge interrupted with the comment that he had already found, as a matter of fact, at an earlier stage of the proceedings that the abuse had occurred. The witness expressed puzzlement at the difference between legal and clinical fact:

> *Expert:* It appears there is a difference between the legal and clinical views of the facts here, Your Honor.
>
> *Judge:* Let me ask it this way. If you assume the sexual abuse is true, does that alter your opinion in the case?
>
> *Expert (struggling to place this hypothetical question into conjunction with his analysis of the case, which led to the opposite conclusion):* Well, Your Honor (slowly and thoughtfully), if the abuse did occur, that would be a different case from the present one, so I guess my opinion would of course be different.
>
> *Judge (triumphantly, as if he had just proved his point):* Right!

Some practitioners respond to this concern with the origins of information by using, or even overusing, the term *alleged,* as in "The patient alleges he has two brothers." It is probably more diplomatic to use the term only for sensitive material (for example,

"The patient alleges that he has a history of antisocial acts."); for routine recording purposes, "states," "reports," or even "says" conveys the necessary source orientation, either in the record or on the witness stand.

# 4

# Types of Witnesses

The usual way in which a psychiatrist might end up in a courtroom is as a fact witness rather than as an expert witness. The role of expert witness is covered in the companion volume, *The Psychiatrist as Expert Witness.* (Please refer to that book for more detailed discussion.)

The essential distinction between the two roles is that the fact witness testifies about matters that he or she has perceived through the senses: seen, heard directly (as opposed to hearsay), touched, tasted, or smelled. Fact witnesses also may, to a limited extent, testify about gestalts that emerge from these immediate observations, such as a syndrome or diagnosis, and about immediate consequences, such as a treatment plan or a therapeutic intervention.

In contrast, an expert witness may draw conclusions from data, including other observers' data; may testify about abstractions, such as the "standard of psychiatric care" in a malpractice case; and may even render opinions about a patient never seen (for example, in a malpractice case about a patient who committed suicide).

As a fact witness, the four typical roles within which you might commonly enter into some form of litigation are as 1) an observer, 2) a treater, 3) a plaintiff, and 4) a defendant. Some representative examples of these fact witness roles follow.

As an observer, you might be a bystander present by happenstance on an inpatient unit, and you might see a fight between someone else's patient and a nurse, or you might observe an interaction involving another patient, nursing staff member, or family member. As an observer type of fact witness, you are a witness in the narrowest focused sense because you just happened to observe (witness) a significant event. A similar sequence of events may bring you into the courtroom setting to report what you saw in the context of some litigation having nothing to do with you.

A common second role for the average psychiatrist is that of treater (more specifically, the nondefendant treater), who has been caring for a patient either *before* a particular claimed injury that has provoked litigation, typically to portray the patient's premorbid state, or *after* a claimed injury to determine the postinjury psychiatric condition in a manner relevant to the claimed damages in the situation. An ethical pitfall concerning testifying about a patient's postinjury psychiatric condition is addressed later in this book in "When Your Patient Sues Someone Else" in Chapter 8.

Third, you might be the plaintiff. You might be suing someone else and might even have grounds to claim your own emotional damages. Using your clinical knowledge, you might describe, as a fact witness, your own symptoms and how they affect your life.

Last, and most regrettably, you might be the defendant against whom the case is brought. For example, as the defendant in a malpractice case in which one of your patients alleges that you did not meet the standard of care, you could state what you saw or observed in this case and what you diagnosed; then, you could report what you did and your rationale for doing it.

To summarize, as a fact witness, you give direct observations, diagnosis, and treatment—what you perceived and did yourself. Essentially, you are reporting narrowly on the results of personal examination of the patient and drawing "conclusions," if any, which adhere closely to those firsthand observations (for example, the patient's diagnosis and prognosis). An ethical tension develops when a fact witness (for example, a treater) is asked to perform the expert witness's role, as reviewed in the next two sections.

## Treater Versus Expert

In general, these two roles—treater and expert—are considered incompatible because the clinical, legal, and ethical mandates are markedly different for them. Because the subject is both important and often confused, I summarize the differences between these two roles in this section, followed by a detailed analysis in the next section and in Appendix 1 to this book.

First, the expert does not traditionally have a physician-patient relationship with the subject of the expert's examination, who is usually called an examinee. Second, the treater's job is to place the patient's welfare first—to help and to heal—whereas the expert's job is, by testimony, to inform and to teach the judge or jury, regardless of whether the expert's testimony helps or harms the patient. The treater's "client" is the patient; the expert's client is the court. The very need of the treater to help the patient constitutes, from a forensic perspective, a form of bias through lack of the requisite objectivity and investment in the outcome.

Additionally, the expert witness is ethically obligated to warn the examinee that the material emerging from the expert's examination is not confidential and might be used in open court in ways that may or may not benefit the patient. In treatment you can usually promise confidentiality, barring emergent circumstances.

Interestingly, psychologists who are members of the American Psychological Association are ethically obliged to give the client an elaborate protocol of warnings in the first session about all of the possible forms of confidentiality breaches, as well as to tell the patient how to go about complaining regarding presumed ethical breaches. Although I have seen no case directly concerning this point, such a protocol would blur the distinction somewhat between clinical and forensic contexts, because, arguably, the psychologists have given a quasi-forensic warning at the outset.

## The Psychotherapist in Court: Some Common Pitfalls

In psychiatric treatment, perhaps especially in the treatment of trauma victims, it is important for the therapist to believe the patient's story of the traumatic experience. The patient will not feel "joined" or understood without this belief. This technical recommendation to treaters extends, of course, far beyond trauma victims as a specific population. One might argue that all good psychotherapists attempt, through the process of empathy, to see the world through their patients' eyes. This deliberate credulousness (similar to the literary "willing suspension of disbelief") permits the empathic immersion in the patient's experience without which much of the therapist-patient rapport is unattainable and successful psychotherapy is compromised. Similarly, such belief often acts as a kind of advocacy for the patient's view, which may aid in mastery of the traumatic experience. In consultative experience, I find a number of common practical, conceptual, and ethical pitfalls occurring for treating therapists who end up in court, most often through failure to understand the distinction between fact witness and expert witness. The nature of these pitfalls and the means of avoiding them are the subject of this discussion.

Why does this issue about fact witness and expert witness even arise? Consultative experience reveals that two types of attorneys most commonly precipitate this conflict: 1) those who simply do not understand the nature of the conflict and the irreconcilable roles of treater versus expert and 2) those who wish to economize by not hiring a separate expert and by deliberately having the treater do "double duty" (this latter group often also fails to understand the nature of the problem). Thus, in practical terms the treater may be subjected to pressure from the patient's attorney (or, rarely, the patient) to change roles or may simply volunteer to serve an expert function out of ignorance or a wish to advocate on behalf of the patient.

## Subjective-Objective Spectrum

An important aspect of the fact-expert dichotomy is that the fact witness's direct observations may be subjective, at least insofar as they are strained through the treater's senses. In contrast, the expert strives for objectivity, which may include paying attention to views opposing those of the patient or discorroborating the latter's claims—two behaviors that would be in ill accord with the treater's role as follows.

The intentional credulousness of the treating therapist is, as previously mentioned, vital. If a patient said, "My mother is a terrible woman," a competent therapist would never reply, "Oh, no, I've met her, and I think she's a fine lady!" The therapist would grasp that the issue in question is the patient's subjective perception, not the mother as she objectively is or the therapist's equally subjective alternative view.

But the same technically valuable credulousness becomes a potential limitation in the courtroom. Treaters are often in danger of failing to appreciate the degree to which their subjective immersion in the patient's experience constitutes an inescapable bias. Especially with trauma victims, therapists are in danger of confusing their therapeutic credulousness with actual knowledge of the external real event or trauma and testifying to that effect.

A specific example is the situation wherein a patient has an exaggerated and idiosyncratic reaction to what might be a minor trauma for the average person. If a patient claims that his or her life was forever changed by a billboard he or she observed or that a fall on the ice shattered forever his or her faith in a benign universe, the therapist accepts this (at least at first) as an emotionally valid description of an experience—an experience that does not necessarily mean that the patient is entitled to damages commensurate with those extreme feelings, even though the patient is entitled to the therapist's compassion. The expert, in contrast, must bring the issue into perspective with reason, fairness, and foreseeability.

## Role Conflict of Interest

A second pitfall on the subjective-objective axis is the failure to perceive what amounts to a conflict of interest between therapist and expert roles. The best way to grasp this issue is to recall the physician's primary admonition, *primum non nocere*—"in the first place, do no harm." The traditional interpretation of this principle is that the physician pledges to do only those things that will help the patient and, by implication, to refrain from all others that might be harmful. This admonition accords reasonably well most of the time with the role of fact witness.

Unfortunately, if pressed into the role of expert and honoring the new mandate of objectivity, the treating psychotherapist may well testify in ways that do not clearly help the patient or may indeed be harmful. Such an outcome necessarily occurs in a context in which the treater has not warned the patient of this potential outcome or of the use to which the material revealed in therapy may be put. This situation poses an ethical bar to the treater functioning as expert. All forensic examinations, by the way, require a warning at the outset of the interview to inform the examinee of whatever limits of confidentiality or other ethical issues may apply to that interview.

## Economic Bias

Another potential pitfall in the treater's serving as expert flows from monetary considerations. Civil litigation usually involves damages. Practically speaking, *damages* means an amount of money considered by the decision maker to represent adequate compensation to the plaintiff for the injury in question. In psychiatric malpractice cases, for example, the money is often earmarked for payment of the therapy that the patient needs to overcome the emotional injuries allegedly caused by the defendant in the case. Under those circumstances, the expert receives only a fee and thus has no financial interest in the outcome of the case; that is as it should be.

The treater, in contrast, *has* a direct financial incentive to be generous at best (or inflationary at worst) in defining the estimated damages, because that money will go directly to the treater to fund the treatment. Although it is theoretically quite possible for a treater to remain free of bias under those circumstances, the appearance of conflict of interest is damaging to the credibility of the plaintiff and hence to the strength of the case, if any.

## Determining the Standard of Care

A central element in malpractice cases is the question of *negligence,* usually defined in terms such as a failure to render care at the level of the average reasonable practitioner. Whether care meets this standard is an expert question or conclusion; depending on jurisdiction, the standard may be determined by regional practice ("locality rule") or national practice as conveyed by national journals and meetings. Focus on the average maintains fundamental fairness; it would be inappropriate to hold all practitioners to the level of the best and fault them for falling below that. A conclusion that an expert might draw in a typical malpractice case is that the care delivered to the plaintiff in the case did or did not meet the standard of care. Most malpractice cases require that the expert demonstrate at some point how he or she has become aware of the standard of care, especially if the expert practices in a different setting. Access to the standard may come to the expert by wide teaching or consultation experience, organizational meetings, conferences, and seminars; peer review activities both for quality of care and for journal articles; and similar sources. This knowledge base validates the expert's opinion.

A pitfall for the treater concerning standard of care is an egocentric view: "The way I do it is the right way, and other ways are below the standard of care." This simplistic formulation misses the pluralistic nature of modern psychiatry.

## Hindsight Bias

*Hindsight bias* is the principle that retrospective vision is 20/20 because the events have already occurred. When the psychotherapist is treating a patient whose previous treater was negligent, it is easy for the current treater to forget that he or she already knows the outcome (by hindsight) of the alleged negligence. However, knowing the outcome by hindsight does not necessarily mean that—in the "foresight view" of the previous treater—the outcome was foreseeable. The legal notion of foreseeability is essential to the finding of negligence: could the harm have been foreseen under ordinary circumstances?

A particularly common pitfall is the subsequent treater's beliefs that his or her present knowledge of the patient is superior to that of the previous treaters, even when the patient earlier had different symptoms or a different condition. Again, the hindsight bias reveals itself: "I know what the outcome is, so I know retrospectively what they should have seen." Such a view is unfair to the previous treaters and slights the real and palpable data—much of it subjective and flowing from being in the actual room and observing the patient before one's eyes—to which a contemporary treater has access.

As it is with diagnosis, so it is with treatment. A subsequent treater must weigh into his or her potential second-guessing of previous therapy the many uncertainties and ambiguities that may have been present then but are now dimmed in the glare of hindsight and knowledge of certain outcomes.

## Goal-Directed Testimony and the Pull of Political Activism

The final pitfall represents a serious confusion of the political with the clinical and legal.

A treating therapist, serving as a plaintiff's expert in a sexual misconduct case, stated (under oath in deposition, incidentally) that she diagnoses all alleged victims of sexual misconduct as suffering from posttraumatic stress disorder, whether or not they meet the criteria, in order to ensure compensation for these patients.

Although one might understand the spirit of such a position, one might also reflect on how such abuse of the diagnostic process may backfire, decreasing the credibility of this expert's testimony to the detriment of the patients.

## Conclusion

Although the courtroom may be perceived as a hostile environment by many clinicians, treating psychotherapists are increasingly called on to enter those precincts and give testimony. This review is intended to highlight common pitfalls for treaters entering into this "foreign country." The major pitfalls addressed in this chapter include differences between fact and expert witnesses, conflicts of roles and interests, subjective and objective viewpoints, foresight and hindsight, and political contamination of the process. Armed with caveats derived from these discussions, the clinician may gain not only increased comfort but also increased effectiveness as a witness in court.

# 5

## Depositions and
## How to
## Survive Them

**A**s a fact witness, it is likely that at some point you may be called for a deposition. Most often this procedure aids *discovery,* the pretrial investigatory process aiding each side in the preparation of its case. The purpose of a deposition is to find out what you will be expected to say at trial, to assess the strength of your testimony and your demeanor and presence as a witness, and at times to preserve your testimony in the event of your unavailability through illness or schedule conflict. This chapter aims to prepare you for what to expect.

## Mechanics of the Deposition

First, the physical setup of a typical deposition takes place at your office or conference room or at the office of one of the attorneys in the case. Location is largely a matter of scheduling and convenience. On some occasions, when the attorneys are from out of town, the office of a local law firm may be used for this purpose.

The players are typically as follows: yourself as the witness; the attorney, usually functioning as "your" attorney, who represents you or your patient; the other attorney(s) in the case representing the party or parties involved; and the stenographer, who, as we shall see, is the most important participant. On occasion, the stenographer will be accompanied by videotape technicians if the deposition is being taped.

In most cases, the attorneys begin by identifying themselves for the record and stating whom they represent. They agree on certain ground rules, called *stipulations,* that need not concern you, and then you are sworn in, meaning the oath to tell the truth is administered to you by the stenographer as you raise your right hand. The language of this oath may vary among jurisdictions, but the intent is the same. The oath is sworn testimony under penalties of perjury. After the oath, the questions usually begin.

You usually will be asked if you wish to read and sign the deposition to check for errors. I recommend that you do this, because minor typographical errors and homophones can create serious misunderstandings (a leading journal recently apologized for a transcription error where the comment "it's an us-and-them situation" was transcribed "it's an S and M situation"). There is also a danger for novice witnesses "zoning out" from anxiety and not really getting the questions.

## Content of the Deposition

A deposition is usually described as an oral examination under oath as part of the discovery process whereby the opposing attorney (usually) asks you questions to discover what you know and what your testimony at trial is likely to be. This straightforward portrayal, however, masks many pitfalls and misperceptions.

First, although it may seem a quibble, a deposition is not an oral examination under oath; it is the *written record* of the oral examination under oath, a fact that has an effect on what the deposition is used for and how you should approach it. For one thing, the information that is written down may be used later to challenge you, catch you in a contradiction, or impeach you.

One important implication of this written record is the need to clarify who your audience is. In the courtroom, it would be the judge—usually a former lawyer—or the jury—usually (although there are exceptions) a group of people with a ninth- through twelfth-grade level of education (once in my life, in Durham, North Carolina, I had a jury in which everyone was a college graduate; it never happened before and it hasn't happened since). Because a deposition is the written record of the oral examination under oath, that means that the audience for the deposition is the *stenographer.* This unexpected conclusion has certain implications for the manner in which you should answer questions. To grasp this point more readily, picture yourself testifying at trial. In that context, you should be testifying—talking—in a friendly manner to the jury, attempting to seem relaxed (whether or not you feel it), and trying to use jargon-free, basic English without any complicated terms or subordinate clauses.

In contrast, in the deposition, you want to do several things. First, there are five answers in a deposition: 1) yes, 2) no, 3) I don't know, 4) I don't recall, and 5) a brief narrative. Regarding the brief narrative, you want to make every effort to ensure that your answer cannot be quoted out of context. You do this by incorporating the question into the answer, despite how deadly dull this makes your answers sound (but remember, it is not the sound that matters; it is the stenographer's written record). Thus, when somebody says, "Do you feel that the standard of care was met in your treatment of this case?" you could simply say, "Yes," but it is far better to say, "I believe my treatment did meet the standard of care because . . . " so that it is much more difficult to quote this answer out of context.

If you disregard this advice and get into the deposition room and start bantering and chatting and having a wonderful time conversing, then you are not being sufficiently protective and careful of the development of the written record of your deposition. This lack of care may hurt you later at trial.

To address this issue in another way, the language in a deposition should be precise, formal, austere, and self-sustaining for the question. In other words, the question should be incorporated so completely into the answer that even when the answer is read out of context, you technically wouldn't need to know what the question was because you could infer or construct it from the answer.

Because the stenographer is your audience, it is important to understand how to save your stenographer's sanity. Some additional tips follow:

- Speak out loud. Don't shrug, nod, or grunt because these gestures don't transcribe accurately.
- Speak in turn. Don't overlap your answer with the question, even if the lawyer is asking a long, ponderous question to which you have long since figured out the answer. Stepping on the other person's speech drives the stenographer crazy trying to write down what both speakers say. Wait for the other person to finish, and don't overlap with his or her conversation.
- Speak slower than usual because the stenographer has to record your answer correctly. Getting back a deposition for review and finding it full of errors because you spoke too fast is annoying and a waste of time and money for everybody.
- Spell the odd words and names of drugs, diagnoses, and technical terms.
- Don't discuss the merits of the case or your views of it with the stenographer. The fact that the stenographer is your audience doesn't mean that he or she is your friend. Keep the relationship professional.
- Give stenographers your business card before you are sworn. The business card is helpful if you have a somewhat unusual or often misspelled name, and the stenographer can contact you if any questions arise about names or technical terms that you used and so on.

The following is a real-life example of a witness not "getting it" when receiving an instruction during a deposition:

> *Question:* . . . and likewise I'll wait for you to finish your answer before I ask my next question. Okay?
> *Answer:* Uh-huh.
> *Question:* Also, if you give verbal answers, rather than nods or shrugs, the court reporter can take that down.
> *Answer:* (Witness moves head in an affirmative response.)

Note how stenographers formally describe nonverbal responses. Even more deliberately neutral records are not uncommon: witness indicating, witness moves head up and down (sideways), or no verbal response. These cumbersome locutions are all in the service of scrupulously avoiding the appearance of imputing a substantive response to a nonverbal gesture.

Other stenographer-centered maneuvers include the following: if you don't understand the question, ask that it be repeated or read back as many times as you need for clarity; turn to face the stenographer without worrying that the questioning attorney will feel you are rude; speak slowly, distinctly, carefully, and in intact sentences; and take your time and rehearse your answer in your mind, looking for possible misunderstandings and distortions that might lie in a particular choice of words. You will surely find that your answers in this form will sound to you cumbersome, slow, affected, pompous, prolix, sententious, and—maybe to your own ears—phony. None of that matters. You are trying to create a solid written record, not communicate to a jury.

## Objections

At various points during your deposition, your attorney may raise objections by stating for the record, "Objection." In some, but not all, cases, the basis may be stated as well, such as "object to form," "objection, [lack of] foundation," or "objection, assumes facts not in evidence." You should pause after each question anyway, to take time to think and to allow for such objections to be made.

In general, objections are "just for the record"; that is, they do not preclude your answering but are designed to affect later admissibility to the trial process of the points under discussion. Occasionally, the attorney may drop the old question and try to coin a better one. Sometimes one or the other attorney may say, "You may answer." Unless your attorney *instructs* you not to answer, go ahead and reply.

You really do not need to worry about the *bases* for any objections, because that is the attorney's problem, not yours. The following is an example from a suicide malpractice case:

> *Physician-witness:* I saw the patient run toward the window on the inpatient unit yelling, "I can't take it any-more!"
> *Attorney:* What was the patient trying to do?
> *Other attorney:* Objection [to form or speculation; as phrased, the question seems to require the physician to read the patient's mind].
> *Attorney (attempting a remedy):* Based on your experience as a psychiatrist, did you entertain any concerns about the patient at that point?
> *Physician-witness:* Yes.
> *Attorney:* What were they?
> *Physician-witness:* I was afraid the patient was making a suicide attempt.

You may hear at some point, "Objection, move to strike!" This remark may sound both startling and scary, but you need not brace yourself for a blow. Further, this comment does not imply that your previous answer is untrue. The attorney is merely flagging that part of the testimony for a future challenge to its admissibility as evidence in the proceedings. Alternatively, the attorney may believe that your answer was not responsive to the question asked, in which case the question will be either repeated or rephrased. The "motion" to strike that testimony may or may not be granted later by the judge. That is neither your problem nor your concern. Continue answering the questions.

## Errors and Pitfalls

Clinicians may make some common errors when first going to a deposition. The first category of error is thinking that the deposition *is* like a trial. You may think (erroneously) that you should use the same casual, relaxed, and basic way of speaking that you would use with the jury. The written record of such an approach, again, may not be sufficiently precise and rigorous to prevent its use to impeach you at trial. Second, at trial there is no need for self-standing answers because the jury heard the question, too.

Alas for simplicity, there is one exception to the above rules: the videotaped deposition, which will be played for the jury in your absence if, for example, for medical or schedule reasons, you cannot travel, you are participating in another trial, or you are about to go on vacation. For such situations, attorneys may decide to videotape you and show the videotape as your testimony. Video-taping does not happen often, but it does require a "gearshift" in your mind: a videotaped deposition *is* the equivalent of a trial in that the audience is no longer the stenographer but the jury, who will be seeing the entire give-and-take dialogue between the attorney and yourself on tape. In this situation, you should pretend that the camera is the jury; look at the camera and talk to the camera in basic juror-friendly, jargon-free English. The videotaped deposition, then, is the exception that proves the rule.

The second category of error is thinking the deposition is *not* like a trial. One aspect of this error is misunderstanding that the deposition is an examination *under oath.* This condition requires serious attention to truth and fact; you cannot just cheerfully make up information, wing it, guess, and distort. You have to tell it like it really is because you are under oath, and the issue of perjury is as explicit in this context as it is anywhere else, as part of the legal process.

Another serious pitfall is assuming that this is "just a deposition," not a trial, and therefore you don't have to prepare as much—perhaps you don't have to prepare at all. Such an attitude is clearly a dangerous one, leaving you vulnerable, at the very least, to damaging cross-examination.

Two leading attorneys were quoted as saying that, in a malpractice case, the goal of the plaintiff's attorney in a deposition of the defendant-physician is to get from that physician an admission of negligence in the basic (or so-called *prima facie*) case (1). If, as a defendant, you needed an additional incentive for vigilance and rigor in listening to the questions and the cautious circumspection of your answers, this maxim would be a powerful one. The following example illustrates a physician's costly loss of attention during an actual deposition:

> During a predeposition conference (a meeting in which the defendant-physicians' attorney prepares them for the actual deposition), I asked both physicians to explain the patient's poor result. The neurosurgeon said, "When these discs protrude and compress down on the nerves, they often damage the nerves by compromising the circulation. You have to use very gentle retraction to move the nerves away to get at the disc material. But sometimes, even with the most gentle retraction, the nerves go into spasm. If we hadn't operated, she would have been a paraplegic. Her problems now are severe, but they had nothing to do with negligence. The damage was done to those nerves by the disc compression before we operated."
>
> His explanation was solid, and the neurosurgeon's demeanor made him a strong witness. But at the deposition a few days later, the plaintiff's attorney asked, "Well, if you did such a good job, why is my client in this terrible condition?" Instead of his previous answer, the neurosurgeon replied, "Either Joey (the orthopedist) or I must have pulled too hard on her nerve roots." To this day, I don't know if that remark was a Freudian slip—or merely a slip of the tongue. But it was too late: That brief loss of concentration and an incredibly poor choice of words forced us to settle the case for $450,000. (2, p. 158)

As an additional point, note that one's professional colleagues, no matter how closely held in the bond of friendship, should be referred to by their professional titles: "Dr. Smith," not "Joey."

## Common Attorney Tactics in Deposition

The well-prepared witness should be aware of some common tactics that plaintiffs' attorneys may use in deposing you; these tactics are used not only to obtain the damaging admission of negligence noted previously but also to achieve other goals to the questioner's advantage—and to your disadvantage. Similar issues bear on your depositions on behalf of your patients. Because your goals alter with your different roles, the attorney asking you questions will be referred to as the "examining attorney," with the understanding that this is usually, but not always, someone on the side of the case opposite to your own or to your patient's.

### "Let's Have a Conversation"

This conversational tactic essentially attempts to conceal the fact that a formal and binding examination under oath is taking place. The examining attorney tries to relax you with chat, comments on the weather, remarks about the local sports teams, and so on. The emotional tone is, "Let's just have ourselves a little chat, Doctor. I'm not going to take up a lot of your valuable time; I have only a few simple questions for you, so just relax." The novice deponent is in danger of being lulled into a posture of relaxed vigilance and casual, offhand responses to queries, forgetting that the written record may be used in later impeachment.

A related conversational pitfall is the *sotto voce* comment, a common element in many conversations. But this type of comment is a dangerous example of "muttering for the record." The witness, struggling to decipher a Xerox copy of a progress note and becoming impatient, may mutter, "I can't make heads or tails of this," "I can't figure out *what* they were doing here," or "I can't make sense of this." In muttering so, however, the witness seems to be impugning the *care,* the delivery of which is recorded in the medical record. A better response would be "I am having some trouble reading this note; have you a clearer copy or an original I could look at?"

## Scrambling the Order

Depositions often but not always proceed in a somewhat logical and hence predictable fashion, beginning with inquiry about your name, address, and social security number, and then exploring material from your credentials or curriculum vitae to get a sense of your background and training, as well as any special competence or experience you may have had relevant to the matter at hand. Only then, after this extensive background review, do the first questions come that are directly related to the present issue.

Knowing that you have thought about your case and talked with your attorney, deposing attorneys may try hard to keep you from telling a coherent, safe story. Examining attorneys may try to throw you off by scrambling the order, beginning almost immediately with major questions such as "What are all your opinions in this case?" or "Now, after this person shot himself on your doorstep, whom did you call first?" For many deponents, such queries have the startling feeling of an ambush and may rattle you, as indeed they are intended to do. Your response, however, should not be impulsive, hasty, or flustered. If surprised in reality, you should buy "composure time" by saying something such as "I'd like to think about that for a moment." You should then pause and collect yourself, frame your response to contain the question, and respond, "Immediately after discovering on my doorstep the tragic death of Mr. Jones, my first action was to. . . . "

## The Rhythm System of Witness Control

Attorneys may try to set a pace or rhythm for the questions and, by invitation, your answers. Often, this approach is coupled with a "lulling series" of questions that psychologically prepare you to expect a certain response, after which a trap is sprung, as in the example that follows:

> *Attorney (briskly):* Doctor, did you beat this patient of
>   yours with a club?
> *Physician:* No.
> *Attorney (fast, almost on top of your answer):* Did you
>   stab him with a knife?
> *Physician (equally fast):* No!
> *Attorney:* Did you shoot him with a gun?
> *Physician:* No!
> *Attorney:* Did you give him medication?
> *Physician:* No—wait—uh, I mean, *yes,* yes, I did.

As you see from the example, by encouraging you to keep up with the flow, as it were, the attorney gets you moving to his or her rhythm, which may be faster than not only your natural rhythm but also your chance to think; therefore, you don't have time to weigh your answers appropriately. You should resist the pressure to clip right along with the examining attorney; instead, sit there and think as long as you need to, until you have the answer organized in your mind, and then turn to the stenographer and give that answer.

Note, for completeness, that sometimes at trial, when your own attorney is asking you questions, getting into a rhythm with your questioner may sometimes be an effective method of conveying confidence or providing routine information. However, this approach should probably not be attempted by the beginner, because it can easily sound awkward, false, or facetious.

## An End Run Around Objections

The nonexamining attorney or attorneys may be placing on record objections to certain questions; as noted earlier in this chapter, usually you will answer the question anyway unless instructed not to do so. At times, the examining attorney will attempt to "get into the back door" by making an end run around the objection, that is, by asking a question only superficially different from the one just asked. Remember to pause for that moment and look at your attorney to see if he or she wants to object again or to give you an instruction.

## Deposition Language

Members of the television audience for the Hill-Thomas hearings before Congress may well have come away with the thought (among others): "Why can't these ex-attorneys ask a decent question?" Apparently, going to law school does not equip one with the ability to ask coherent questions; those ex-lawyers, now legislators, seemed incapable of asking a relevant, rational question in terms of organization, structure, and logical coherence of the English language.

The following is an actual question I was asked during a deposition:

> Was that explanation amplified in any way with any details as to what that sexual abuse was supposedly to consist of during that conversation?

Such a query calls for only one possible response: "Could you please rephrase that question?" or "I'm sorry, I didn't understand that." Don't even try to answer this kind of question; whatever your answer, there will be no way to tell what either of you meant.

Witnesses as well are not immune from a case of the arglebargles. A real-life example follows:

> *Question:* Have these symptoms [of posttraumatic stress disorder] been bolstered by research in biological abnormalities in the brain?
>
> *Answer:* Yes. This is a summary of some of the 1994 article by van der Kolk, "Biological Abnormalities in PTSD."
>
> *Question:* Could you break that down into understand-able—

*Answer:* Yes, the psychophysiology. We've been
talking a lot about that. As a clinician, that's the
thing that you see. A lot of these other things
are dependent upon blood studies, serum from
spinal fluid, other kinds of research; methodol-
ogy, much of it on Vietnam veterans and much
of it carried on in Yale; in Connecticut, at the
veterans hospital there; a lot of it being carried
on at—in New York; and a lot of it carried on in
Boston. Okay. Extreme autonomic arousal remi-
niscent of the trauma. You know, I sort of described—I think I described that one. One that
gets us here is what we call the neurotransmit-
ters, and what we have found—there is an alarm
system in the brain—and I'm going to show you
that—but basically what happens is the norad-
renergic system, which is noradrenaline that
comes within the brain from the spinal cord,
and epinephrine that you know about, comes
from the gland on the kidney. I can't—I've got a
blind spot here.

The "blind spot" here is the witness's complete loss of perspective taking. Apparently reading from some written material not
identified in sufficient detail or without sufficient quotation marks
to follow, the witness is reading a bit, commenting a bit, editorial-
izing a bit, tossing in the odd verbal footnote, addressing the attorneys a bit to remind them of previous points—the result being an
essentially incoherent record.

An additional difficulty is posed by questions including double
negatives. These questions come in a wide variety, but the common factor for the deponent is the fact that the same answer may
be either accurate or the *opposite* of accurate (in this regard,
such questions resemble the have-you-stopped-beating-your-
wife school of inquiry where either "yes" or "no" is equally in-
criminating).

Here is an example:

*Attorney (to defendant in sexual misconduct malpractice case):*
But you *never* had sex with him, *isn't* that correct? (Emphasis
is added to show double negatives.)

To this query, "yes," "no," or even "maybe" would confuse this
issue rather than clarifying it, as in that classic line, "Yes, we have
no bananas." "Yes" in this context could mean "Yes, I did have sex"
as well as "No," that is, "You are correct, I did not." "No" could
mean "I *did* have sex, so no, you are *in*correct" or "Yes, I never
did."

The only useful response would be either to request a rephrase
of the question or actively rephrasing the core point in your answer yourself: "It is correct to say I never had sex with him." Note
also that your rephrase effectively precludes a later jury's misunderstanding your answer if quoted out of context.

## Getting You to Guess

In normal conversation, your companion might ask, "Isn't Smith
the chief executive officer of Widget Manufacturing?" You might
not know at all or might not be sure, but to keep the conversation
going, you might reply, "I think so, why?" And the conversation
would continue. In casual conversation, no harm is done, even
when you give an answer of which you were uncertain. However,
if you guess at an answer during a deposition, you not only may
delight the other side's attorney but also may have to eat your answer in public on cross-examination at trial. Most often, the problem is the basic human fear of looking foolish by not knowing
something you think you should know or you think "they" think
you should know. Here is the drill: even if you think you should
know or it's *usually* so, do not guess. The following example illustrates why:

*Deposing attorney:* And when evaluating a patient, it
would be customary to take a history, correct?
*You:* Yes.

*Deposing attorney (confidently):* Dr. Smith, your colleague did that?
*You (feeling the pressure to support Smith and rea-
   soning that he probably did it—hell, he must
   have done it):* I believe so (although you don't
   know).

At trial, you are made to look silly because the patient came into
the clinic mute and catatonic, but you have inadvertently set the
standard of care for your colleague to fail. "I don't know," "I am
not sure," or "I am not clear on how that works" are perfectly good
answers when true. A similar good answer is, "I don't recall, but if
you want to call my attention to something, I'll be glad to look at
it." If the attorney shows you, you get to see the source; if not, the
attorney looks bad, as if he or she were trying to conceal something.

## The Danger of Conversational Interjections

Consider the following example of deposition dialogue:

*Attorney (appearing to set up a review of the facts):* So,
   you have this 24-year-old man . . .  (attorney speaks
   in an are-you-with-me tone, hesitates, and looks at
   witness as if for confirmation).
*Witness (tentatively, encouragingly, with rising inflec-
   tion):* R-i-i-i-ght . . .
*Attorney:* . . . who goes into the hospital . . .
*Witness (in a keep-talking tone):* R-i-i-i-ght . . .
*Attorney:* . . . and receives negligent treatment . . .
*Witness:* R-i-i-i-ght . . .
*Attorney:* . . . and then is discharged into the commu-
   nity . . .
*Witness:* R-i-i-i-ght . . . (and so on).

This kind of dialogue must occur countless times in informal
settings: the storytellers check to see if their audience is with

them, and the listeners send various socially sanctioned verbal and nonverbal signals (such as right, wow, you don't say, uh-huh, yeah, a nod) to convey ongoing attention and reassure speakers of continued interest. In this example, however, the written transcript is stripped of all this interpersonal and nonverbal "music" of tone and glance. The remaining bare words contain the witness's acknowledgment, almost in passing, that negligent treatment occurred ("Right"), without the apparent realization that this wheel-greasing conversational interjection has essentially conceded the case to the other side. In such a situation, the witness should simply wait quietly until the entire question is out or respond "I'm listening" until the time to give a full answer.

## Personal Questions

Attorneys may ask personal questions as legitimate elements of discovery. Asking your date of birth, for example, provides not only your age but also some sense of career milestones, your experience in the field, or your seniority. Even some quite personal questions arguably may have a direct relevance, such as whether you are a recovering alcoholic, when the issue is your treatment of a patient with a similar condition.

Unfortunately, attorneys also may ask totally inappropriate and intrusive personal questions simply to rattle you. Examples include your total income, the grounds for your divorce, your mental health history, or the mental health history of family members. The problem with such questions lies in part in the fact that there is no judge present to rule on their relevance and thus to protect you. Remember that you do not have to answer such questions if they genuinely have nothing to do with the case; indeed, a good answer to such an inquiry is, "I choose not to answer that question, but I assert that my marital status has no impact on my testimony in this case."

The attorney who is "more nearly on your side," such as the patient's attorney, does not represent you and thus cannot tell you that you need not answer or instruct you not to answer. If you choose not to answer, deposing attorneys may threaten to take the matter to a judge to compel your disclosure; let them do so. In such a situation, your own attorney can be helpful as your representative and protector; you may even request a recess and call from the deposition to receive guidance. If indeed a judicial order is ultimately produced compelling some testimony, answer that question.

## Reading and Signing

When the deposition is finished, you have the right to read and sign it. After the stenographer has transcribed the record into a stapled or bound booklet (copies of which are sent to all the attorneys), you may either review and correct this manuscript or waive this privilege, trusting the stenographer's accuracy.

Despite my admiration for the skill of almost every stenographer I have met, I strongly recommend reading and signing. There are too many possible chances for honest errors and sound-alike words or phrases to pass up this opportunity. Note that the reading is a chance to proofread testimony, not to change it in any profound way. However, an omitted "not" or a recording of "appropriate" when you said "inappropriate" represents significant misconstructions of your testimony. Note also that this review is an excellent learning experience because you can observe how you answered questions and consider how you might have answered better or differently.

The deposition is accompanied by an errata sheet, a separate page on which you record the page and line of the error and your corrections. This sheet, together with the signature page (on which your signature is usually notarized), is returned to the examining attorney and distributed to the others. For convenience, some signature pages need not be notarized but are simply signed under pains and penalties of perjury. Ask your attorney about this.

# A Model Instruction[1]

The following dialogue is a model of an attorney's introduction to a deposition (all names in the example are fictitious). For completeness and thoroughness, you will be hard pressed to find its match.

> *Attorney:* Good morning, Mr. Jones. My name is Jane Doe. I'm from Doe, Doe, and Roe, and I represent the plaintiff, Susan Green, in a case that's been brought up against you, as well as other defendants. I trust you've had an opportunity to review that complaint and you are familiar with it.
>
> *Deponent:* Certainly.
>
> *Attorney:* I'm going to go through some basic instructions with you before we commence the deposition to make sure that you are clear about what the proceeding is all about. This is a deposition in which I, as well as other attorneys, have the opportunity to ask you questions pertaining to issues involved in this lawsuit. It is extremely important that you understand my question. If you don't understand my question, I'll ask that you tell me so; otherwise, we'll assume that you understood my question and that your answer is responsive to it. Even though we're seated here in your lawyer's office, this is the same as though you were testifying in court.
>
> *Deponent:* Sure.
>
> *Attorney:* You've been sworn to tell the truth, the whole truth, and nothing but the truth, and that's what we all expect. On one hand, if you do not know the answer to a question, it is perfectly acceptable to say that you do not know or do not recall. On the other

---

[1]Model instruction courtesy of Beth Baldinger, Esq.

hand, if you do have some information, I will ask
that you give me what information you have that is
responsive, to the best of your ability, to my questions. Do you understand these instructions?

*Deponent:* I understand.

*Attorney:* It is also very common for a witness or party
to understand what it is that I'm asking and start to
answer before I am finished. Please wait for me to
finish asking my question completely before you begin to respond because the reporter can only take
down one person speaking at a time.

*Deponent:* Okay.

*Attorney:* It's also very common to say uh-huh and nod
your head. While here in the room we all understand, that is not translatable for the court reporter.
You must say yes, no, and answer everything verbally. Do you understand that?

*Deponent:* Yes.

*Attorney:* It's fine if you use a gesture, just make sure
you speak verbally. In the event that any of your attorneys or you hear an attorney in this room raise an
objection to any of the questions, please do not answer my question. Please allow the attorneys the opportunity to put their objections on the record.
You're instructed and directed to answer all of my
questions unless your attorney instructs you otherwise. Do you understand that?

*Deponent:* Yes.

*Attorney:* Do you have any questions of this proceeding
before we begin today?

*Deponent:* No, I don't.

As a final point, remember that if the tension gets too high and
you need a moment to regroup when you are feeling pressured,
you can always take a break; you are also permitted to ask for
breaks to get water or coffee, use the rest room, or make time-
sensitive calls. If there will be a planned interruption, such as tele-

phone calls, it is courteous to inform the examining attorneys at the outset so that they can pace themselves.

## Conclusion

Depositions are serious business, but paying attention to the principles in this chapter will go far to cushion the blows. Careful preparation both with your attorney and by yourself, coupled with attentive concentration during the proceedings, will lead to your survival.

## References

1. Fuchsberg A, Douglas PJ: Deposing the defendant doctor. Professional Negligence Law Reporter 7:193–194, 1992
2. Griffith JL: Why defensible malpractice cases have to settle. Medical Economics, July 10, 1995, pp 153–158

# 6

## The Trial Itself

Trials hold a terror for most physicians that is driven by movies, television, and the awesome power of our own fantasies. Yet some knowledge and preparation can go a long way toward allaying some of the more gratuitous fears. Remember that the witnessing itself—the observations you made or treatment you provided—has already happened and is in the past. The testifying that now lies ahead is a kind of teaching to laypersons (judge and jury) about what you saw and did. As with other "tough audiences"—uninterested students, resistant patients—the setting is adversarial, but none of its challenges is insurmountable, and at least one attorney in the room is on your side.

Some of the techniques and concepts that you have already learned for depositions will aid you in facing the stresses of trial (and it *is* stressful for almost all the parties involved, as is discussed later in this chapter). Some approaches will have to be altered or modified to fit the new context. In this chapter, I aim to prepare you for your appearance at trial. For the purposes of *this* book, your designated role is a fact witness who knows certain information considered to be relevant to the case at hand. As a result of this specific role, you will be spared the necessity of defending your credentials and conclusions in the same manner as would the expert witness in court.

Later in this book (see "A Nervous Trot Through the Law" in Chapter 8), I place the trial in its context and sequence for a malpractice proceeding. You may wish to refer back to the following discussions at that point.

## Six Ps of Trial Preparation

Preparing for trial is a complex and often strenuous process, even if you are not the defendant-physician in a malpractice case. This preparation can be organized around six principles: preparation, planning, practice, pretrial conference, pitfalls, and presentation.

1. *Preparation:*  Preparation, of course, is the basic element. You should gather all the information and review it for rapid, clear memory access. Review the case, review the chart, review your notes, and get all of the available material up front and at your fingertips.
2. *Planning:*  Recall that courtroom appearances involve both time and stress. Be sure to clear enough time; courts are notoriously unreliable as to scheduling, despite what you may have heard about accommodating physicians' schedules. Plan with your attorney when you will arrive at the courthouse, and arrange for transportation and adequate coverage of your practice, so that you won't be worried or preoccupied. Take care of yourself by not undertaking new projects or seeing new patients; instead, arrange for rest and reflection time, enjoyable activities, and recreation. Resist the temptation just to take your courtroom appearance in stride.
3. *Practice:*  Although there is much about a trial that you cannot predict, the facts of the case and your consequent direct testimony will usually be more predictable. Do not be shy about

practicing your testimony in front of your attorney or even a friend who can give you feedback as to whether you sound clear and confident. Rehearse several different ways of making your main points, and select those that seem clearest to your rehearsal audience.

4. *Pretrial conference:*   It is essential that you meet (either in court or at the lawyer's or your own office the night before) with "your" attorney immediately before you go on the stand to find out what new facts or issues have come out or what the tone is in the courtroom into which you will be thrust. Do not accept evasion of this meeting. Some attorneys are surprisingly casual about this. Such an attorney will typically say, "Well, we're going on at 9:00 A.M., so why not come by the courthouse around oh, say, 8:53. We'll have a cup of coffee; we'll chat." You must emphatically say, "I'm sorry, that's unacceptable. I'll meet with you at 8:00 in the morning in the courtroom conference room (or 7:30 P.M. in your office the night before), and we'll review my testimony so I'll be better prepared for what I'm getting into."

5. *Pitfalls:*   Being alert to the pitfalls at trial means knowing in advance 1) the weaknesses or limits of your testimony and 2) any critical legal point or precise statutory language on which some issue in the case may turn. In anticipation of cross-examination, such pitfalls can be explored by asking yourself the following questions: What will the opposing attorneys try to get me to say? Where are the hot spots, the weak spots, the ambiguities in the case? What are the historical or evidentiary pitfalls? What are the skeletons in my own closet that might be used to impeach me by innuendo (that embarrassing marijuana bust in high school, that arrest for picketing the nuclear plant)? Although this strategy is really up to your lawyer, students of jury decision making recommend that any such pitfalls or weaknesses should be brought up directly; if they are later brought out during cross-examination, you can say, "I've already addressed that issue," thereby stealing the opposition's thunder (1).

6. *Presentation:*   It is not enough that you know what happened

because it's your case and you have reviewed it so intensely. You also must consider how you are going to present this largely technical material to a lay audience of nonpsychiatrists. How are you going to make clear to them your clinical judgment, your reasoning, and most of all, your underlying caring for the patient expressed in your delivery of care? Both preparation and practice are subsumed in presentation.

The six Ps are relevant for observer, treater, or plaintiff, but they are particularly critical if you are the defendant. Several specific issues relevant to your appearance in court are reviewed in the following discussions.

## Preparing Your Attorney

What should be *your* role in preparing your attorney for the upcoming litigation? I use the term *your attorney* because he or she might be your personal attorney when you are being sued for malpractice, or he or she might be the attorney for whose side you are testifying (for example, your patient's attorney if your patient, as plaintiff, is claiming some emotional harms). In any case, it will be necessary for you to educate your attorney by explaining the clinical (that is, psychiatric) issues of the case. These might include diagnosis, psychotherapy, psychopharmacology, indications for hospitalization, and so on.

For some attorneys, this task is barely an issue, simply because from trial experience they know more psychiatry than do many psychiatrists in the United States. Other attorneys are starting more nearly from scratch and may require extensive educating. Do not begrudge this time or attempt to delegate the task to the expert witnesses, if any, on the case; it is time well spent by you and you alone. A properly prepared attorney is your best ally in court.

Demystification is also quite helpful. Many laypersons, including attorneys who are not familiar with psychotherapy, for example, may view it as something of a voodoo science, full of arcane terminology and mystical activities. Demystification may be needed over and above simple education.

Next, you can educate your attorney as to the limits of the data. An attorney may not fully grasp that symptoms and history are fundamentally self-reports; only rarely does the psychiatrist have external evidence for the facts related. You may need to explain that the patient's report is not proof. Moreover, there are limits to the amount of independent corroboration you can obtain without losing the therapeutic alliance.

Finally, a challenging part of attorney preparation is your own awareness and alertness to various pressures and seductions that accompany going to court. You need to be alert to the fact that there will be time pressures to develop opinions before all the data are in, patient pressures to give favorable testimony, and seductions—monetary, narcissistic, and others—aimed at trying to convince you to do or say various things. Psychiatrists working closely with attorneys report how a growing identification with the attorney and with the attorney's position is a natural concomitant of the close working relationship. It is critical to keep this relational phenomenon from biasing your testimony. The issue transcends perjury, becoming an ethical mandate: the truth, the whole truth, and nothing but the truth, including the limits of data and areas of ignorance.

## Dressing for Success

A surprisingly important issue is how you dress. Lecture audiences occasionally balk when I make this point, arguing that giving any weight to how you dress is unfair, unjust, petty, shallow, and ultimately irrelevant to your knowledge and professional skills. Some audience members sputter, "But—a turtleneck sweater—that's who I am!" My response is, perhaps so, but in the real world of the courtroom, in the glare of attention, you want every advantage you can obtain, every nuance in your favor—including how you appear.

To grasp this issue, consider what might be called "Chanel's law," quoted by designer Coco Chanel in a recent movie. The quote (I cannot vouch for its accuracy or authenticity, but it captures the point perfectly) is: "Dress shabbily, they notice the dress; dress impeccably, they notice the woman." To make the point clearer, anything that calls attention to your mode of dress or personal ornamentation is a distraction from what you have to say and, therefore, a bad idea. The implication is that the least-distracting mode of dress is conservative, although, for your comfort, it should be comfortably old and "broken in" (do *not* buy new shirts for appearing in court).

Men and women should dress essentially like the lawyers they see in court and in the media. For men, a suit and tie are preferable because in some parts of the United States, a sports jacket, turtleneck, or the absence of a tie may connote an excessively casual attitude or even disrespect. Women should avoid dresses, pants, and shorts, as well as high-heeled shoes and flats. Stick with the business suit and the medium-heel business shoe, and you will not go wrong.

Avoid ostentation. Leave the $3,000 diamond-studded Rolex watch at home, and wear the rubber Timex in court; avoid elaborate dangling earrings, dramatic jewelry, multiple bracelets and chains, and electric colors. (A wonderful example of the effect of dress on attention occurs in the John Waters movie *Serial Mom* with Kathleen Turner. In one of the scenes in which she is defending herself at trial, Kathleen Turner is so distracted by the fact that one of the jurors has committed the fashion gaffe of wearing white shoes after Labor Day that she loses her entire train of thought.)

In addition to dressing conservatively, keep in mind that you should turn off beepers and cellular telephones when you go to court, and arrange for suitable coverage so that you will not be interrupted. Jurors are commonly annoyed at these interruptions during testimony (and may interpret them as arrogant demonstrations of how busy and important you think you are), but I have known judges to become enraged: the electronic intrusion is seen as disrespect of the court, which is perilously close to contempt. A word to the wise . . . .

After you are suitably attired, with beeper turned off, the next step is taking the witness stand. The most important principles are examined in the following sections.

## Deposition Language
## Versus Trial Language

In your deposition, the stenographer was the most important party and constituted your audience, because he or she was preparing your written record, the essence of the deposition. In keeping with this fact, your deposition answers were designed to be question-containing, short, austere yet complete, and well aimed at the stenographer. In the trial, in contrast, your audience is the jury or judge. In this arena, *what* you say is almost less important than *how* you say it. For example, there may be occasions when a slightly *less* precisely accurate explanation for how something works may be preferable if it is more understandable to a lay jury audience.

In keeping with this change in audience, if you are asked a question at trial, answer that question until you have made your point to completion. Take as long as you need. If someone grows impatient and rudely interrupts you, your credibility is unaffected, because you are the person who has been interrupted while trying to give testimony, and everyone gets mad at, or suspicious of, the attorney. If someone says, "Tell us how you understood the patient's problem," answer that question until you are completely through.

There are, of course, some limits to this approach (there are only so many days allotted for a trial), and you certainly don't want to put the jury to sleep. Indeed, the slightest hint of jury squirming or the dreaded "eye-glaze" sign is cause for bringing your discourse to a speedy resolution.

Another kiss of death during trial testimony occurs when you as the witness do not sound particularly interested in what you are saying. This situation can create an unspoken juror mentality such as "Look, you're actually involved in this case and I'm just a juror; why should I be interested if you're not?"

# Graphics and the Blackboard

As mentioned earlier in this chapter, the essential function of the physician as witness is to teach; hence, a tremendous benefit accrues from skillful use of graphics and the blackboard or flip chart. These devices have certainly been helpful in most lecture-style teaching, but the reason these methods are particularly effective in the courtroom is because of what might be called the paracommunication effect.

Laypersons, including jurors, may harbor all kinds of feelings about physicians in general; such feelings are variations on the theme of transference, influenced by actual previous experience with internists, pediatricians, and gynecologists, as well as mental health professionals. Although your demeanor on the witness stand will be the ultimate determinant of the jury's reaction to you, most juries have generally positive feelings about physicians; however, some might have negative ones. Among these negative feelings, a common one is that physicians don't talk to their patients enough or reveal enough of their decision making as it affects their patients' welfare. In court, you will be doing exactly this: talking to the jury and explaining your reasoning. Properly handled, this explaining can be gratifying to jurors and can give them a break from the talking-heads monotony of the trial.

In addition, when you pick up a piece of chalk in your hand and you stand in front of the blackboard, you become, as a transference object, the most trusted figure in common human experience: the teacher. The teacher *knows.* The juror may not know what the capital of Virginia is—or what chlorpromazine is used for—but knows the teacher knows. The power of this image transcends what you actually draw; what counts is the apparent effort to get your point across, because juries respond to the idea that you are *trying* to help them understand. Thus, whenever it may clarify a point, don't hesitate to use the blackboard or flip chart. Using these devices and what you will draw or list should be reviewed with your attorney in advance, of course, to permit the attorney's intelligent exploration of the issue.

## Time to Testify

What about testifying itself? When asked a question, pause just a moment before answering. This brief delay permits you to replay the question in your head, ensures that you understand it, and allows your attorney to object if desired. That momentary pause is really important; you may not even have to answer the question if the objection is sustained. To keep the jury clear on what is happening, try to look thoughtful while you are thinking or even say—if you have to think about the answer a bit—"Well, I'd like to take just a moment to think about that." This statement keeps the jury from interpreting your silence as utter bafflement or as that you dozed off in midtrial—neither view redounding to your credit or credibility.

No one is usually bothered when you ask for time to think—you won't "look dumb" for having to do so—because it shows that you are taking your testimony seriously.

## The Words You Say

The most vital tightrope you must walk during your trial testimony is the one stretched between being clear and being patronizing. Your use of basic, jargon-free English is absolutely essential, yet you must never talk down (or even seem to talk down) to the jury. One of my colleagues, testifying on "Court TV," said to the jury of a criminal trial, "My job was to disconfirm the hypothesis"; that would be totally over the heads of almost all juries.

Why are your words so important? You might lose the jury for a moment or two, but you can eventually clear up any misunderstandings, can't you? In fact, the answer is no. There *is* an opportunity for redirect examination; however, the issue is not just a matter of dealing with the jury's lack of understanding. Going over the jury's head is alienating and antagonizing, and you may be given no chance to recover the jury's good opinion.

How should you handle technical terms? Is there some way to

explain *dysthymia* without using that term? How do you describe borderline personality disorder to a jury when some psychiatrists don't even understand it? Practice with a critical audience goes a long way to assist you in finding a way to express these complex ideas in simple, but not overtly and obviously simplistic, ways.

If, despite your good intentions and conscientious rehearsal, you find yourself lapsing into jargon, define the term after you use it without making too big a deal of it. Explain terminology as part of your narrative, and don't make a production of explaining it:

Wrong:

*Witness (pompously):* Upon careful and meticulous observation, I made the diagnosis of dysthymia; now, you probably don't know what that means, and why should you? It is a term that we trained psychiatrists use to describe what the ordinary mortal would term a depression lasting . . .

Better:

*Witness:* I thought my patient was suffering from dysthymia, a long lasting depression, and I . . .

Note that the description of dysthymia is a bit casual but not wrong; if it is important to fill in the details, that question will be asked later. The point here is that a bit of jargon that crept in was smoothly defined in an offhand, nonpatronizing manner.

During the previously mentioned "momentary pause," it is a given that you will think before you speak. As a concomitant of this idea, don't shoot from the hip and don't trip on your own ego, especially in thinking that you know it all. A common example of shooting from the hip is when you really don't know the answer but you are willing to guess or to speculate by extrapolation from your usual procedure, for example. Resist this temptation. This practice is extremely dangerous. It is far better to say, "I don't know" or "I don't recall," even if you fear that will make you sound foolish. That is a far sounder position to be in than having to retract that guess or speculation on cross-examination when the inquiring attorney is not your ally.

In court you are, of course, aware of the plaintiff and the defendant and who is who, but recall that those terms are depersonalized. As a rule you should *not* refer to the parties by those names. You want to express yourself in vivid, functional terms: "My patient, Mrs. Jones" (not "the plaintiff"); "I consulted Dr. Johnson" (not "my codefendant"). If you think you can get away with it, you might even want to say "poor Mrs. Jones" to convey your sympathy: she is a suffering person, not just a pawn in the legal game. Be careful with this locution; it could sound sarcastic, especially if the patient is on the other side of the case from you. Never, however, use patients' first names; this will either sound demeaning or excessively intimate, neither of which aids your presentation. Use last names and honorifics even if, in reality, you were always on a first-name basis with the patient.

## Pitfalls and Hot Spots

Although experience is inevitably the best teacher of how to handle trial testimony, there are some points that might stave off the more egregious difficulties.

### Witness Fees

As is the case in psychotherapy and billing practices, money can be a sensitive issue on the witness stand. Fact witnesses are usually paid no fee for their time or a token "subpoena fee" (for example, in Massachusetts, this is a generous $8.00 one-time honorarium). Their participation as witnesses in the judicial system is considered part of their civic responsibility, like jury duty. If you are the treating psychiatrist testifying on behalf of your patient, you are free to negotiate a fair rate with your patient; occasionally, an attorney will agree to pay you an expert hourly fee, despite your fact witness role, even though the rationale for doing so is pretty flimsy. If this arrangement will govern, get something in writing about it before trial. Because of the clinical and ethical conflicts involved (see Chapter 4 in this volume), you should not attempt to solve this problem by functioning as an expert if you are already the treater. Whatever arrangement is made, acknowledge it frankly on the stand.

## "Never" and "Always"

Predictably, the terms *never* and *always* are land mines disguised as ordinary words. They also could be described as empty sets, because few things in psychiatry, at least, are never or always true. You will not go wrong if you regard any question containing these terms as a trap. Use them sparsely if at all in your own testimony.

## Misquotation of Your Testimony

Inaccurate or slightly distorted quotes of your previous testimony are a common ploy. For example, if the opposing attorney says, "Doctor, do you remember before when you testified that physicians were free to abuse every patient they see?" you might say, "I have to admit, counselor, although that doesn't sound familiar to me, I do recall commenting on how difficult it was for physicians to police themselves." Just because the attorney begins a query with your previous testimony does not mean that what comes out is really what you said; the lawyer is not under oath. Assuming automatically that the lawyer is quoting you accurately is dangerous.

## Subordinate Clauses as a Foot in the Door

Examine another technical point that may be useful in giving complete testimony. Assume for the moment that your answer, in the previous example, omitted the "although." Thus: "I have to admit, counselor, that doesn't sound familiar to me." You then draw in your breath to continue with "I do recall . . . ," but at this point, the attorney would be within his or her rights to interrupt you and say, "That's all right if you don't remember what you said, Doctor, you've answered the question, and the record will speak for itself." Note how this latter version makes you seem to have a poor memory at best or to wish to retract sworn testimony at worst. By beginning your answer with a subordinate clause (that is, "although that doesn't sound familiar to me, I do recall . . . "), you effectively compel the questioner to wait for the end of the completed answer, lest he or she seem to be interrupting you.

## Simple Harassment

An old saying attributed to Marcus Tullius Cicero exhorts lawyers to this effect: "When the facts are in your favor, argue the facts; when the facts are not in your favor, yell and pound on the table." My own experience suggests that as a witness you have less to fear from the screaming table pounders than from the soft-spoken, scrupulously polite, cherubic choirboys that lead you down the garden path without your realizing it.

Fortunately, for you as witness, lawyer harassment tends to occur far less often than television and movies would suggest. Lawyers are actually concerned with seeming to be too harsh toward the witness, and judges are usually pretty sensitive as well to the occasional need for "protection" of the fact witness. In fact, despite the ever-popular courtroom drama cliché wherein the attorney is screaming abusive questions to the cowering witness's face from a range of 6 inches, most of the time lawyers are not even allowed to approach you on the witness stand without both good cause and the judge's permission.

Nonetheless, you should be prepared for harassment, with the explicit goal of not letting it touch you at all. Let it bounce off, the way that you may do when a borderline patient is screaming at you that you are an incompetent therapist. It has nothing to do with you or your testimony. Moreover, maintaining your cool has a positive effect on your presentation before the jury. Conversely, of course, losing your cool has the opposite effect.

## Impugning Your Pretrial Preparation

Attorneys may attack you for your preparation prior to trial: "Doctor, isn't it true that you met with your attorney just before appearing on this stand?" The idea behind this query is that you are somehow being coached and that your testimony is inauthentic. The truthful response is always best. You might respond, "Of course, I did; I insist on meeting with my attorney because that's what my lawyer is for—to help me understand these proceedings."

## Nonblissful Ignorance

Most psychiatrists cherish a deep resistance to admitting on the witness stand that they do not understand a question or do not know an answer; like other resistances, this one must be overcome. Do not be afraid to say, "I don't understand the question" or "I don't know the answer to that." It is the lawyer's job to ask you a question in a form or a manner that you can understand; if you don't, the attorney should rephrase the question or ask something else. Similarly, no one remembers everything. If an attorney needs you to recall something for subsequent queries, he or she may show a document.

If you don't recall a fact needed to answer a question, but you know where to look it up in the medical records in front of you on the witness stand, it is appropriate to offer, "I don't recall that, but I think I can find it in just a moment." If it is critical, most attorneys will let you look it up. They also may show you a blowup of the chart or make a representation about the point (a *representation* means that the attorney is supplying the missing fact in order to move on to the next question); for example: "Doctor, let me represent to you that the August 1st discharge summary gives a final diagnosis of schizophrenia. Would it surprise you then to learn . . . ?"

Remember that if you really do not recall, do not guess or infer. If the point is important, the lawyer is obligated to find it and show it to you so that you can give a valid answer.

## The Patient's Presence

Even when your patient is the litigant, he or she may not be at all times present in the courtroom. If the patient is present, respectful language should be maintained with utmost care. You do not want to say, "I diagnosed Mr. Jones as a typical common thug of the born-loser variety" (2, p. 370). You want to say, instead, "Mr. Jones gave me a long history of antisocial acts and incarcerations." The approach of objectivity is best achieved by stating the simple facts.

# Conclusion

Even for the trial-seasoned witness, going to court is rarely an unalloyed pleasure. Some familiarity with the overt and latent issues and some introduction to the useful techniques discussed in this chapter may at least mitigate the more traumatic aspects.

# References

1. Williams KD, Bourgeois MJ, Croyle RT: The effects of stealing thunder in criminal and civil trials. Law and Human Behavior 17:597–609, 1993
2. Appelbaum PS, Gutheil TG: Clinical Handbook of Psychiatry and the Law, 2nd Edition. Baltimore, MD, Williams & Wilkins, 1991

# 7

## Writing for Court

**W**riting reports for use in legal matters is a common practice for expert witnesses. This subject is discussed further in the companion volume, *The Psychiatrist as Expert Witness.* In the ordinary course of psychiatric practice, however, the occasion may arise to communicate with courts or with comparable regulatory bodies such as licensing agencies and registries of motor vehicles. Such communications may include various letters of permission or clearance, affidavits, and similar communications. In this chapter, I discuss some important points to keep in mind when this activity intrudes on clinical work.

Note in general that courts are not particularly interested in spontaneous, unsought input ("As a citizen, let me just point out what's wrong with your approach, Judge Ito"). A court will usually request some specific written input (or solicit your participation in other ways) when it relates to a patient of yours who has become embroiled somehow in the legal system. For example, a patient with chronic schizophrenia, whom you have been treating for several years, has blundered delusionally into someone's house. He has been caught by police and charged with breaking and entering (note, incidentally, that it is quite common for police, on realizing that they are dealing with a psychiatric patient, to take him or her straight to a psychiatric hospital, without even bothering with an arraignment). The patient's public defender asks you to write a letter to the court describing the patient's illness so that the defender can get the case dismissed and the patient transferred to psychiatric care.

## Introductory Data

In the first sentences of the letter, you should establish who you are and what your standing is, that is, how it happens that you are writing to this busy court (almost all courts are busy—a powerful argument to keep all communications short). Here is an example:

> To whom it may concern:
>
> My name is Sigmund Krankheit, M.D. I am a physician specializing in psychiatry and licensed in the Commonwealth of Massachusetts.

The generic form of address is most suitable if the request has not come directly from the judge; if it has, write to that judge by name (for example, Judge William Smith, Middlesex Superior Court). I recommend using the somewhat longer phrasing (rather than "I am a psychiatrist") because even judges sometimes fail to grasp the difference between psychologist and psychiatrist. You should comment on your licensure, perhaps even board certification, but resist the temptation to squeeze in more of your curriculum vitae.

> I am writing at the request and with the permission of Mr. John Jones, . . .

This particular locution emphasizes both that your contribution has been solicited and that the confidentiality barrier has been lifted by the patient himself so that questions of privilege and disclosure have been addressed. If the patient refuses permission, do not reveal data until this matter is cleared up by the court; for example, a court order to disclose information almost always should be honored.

> . . . who is before your court on a charge of breaking and entering (giving the docket number, if you know it, is another time-saver).

This statement identifies the relevance of the patient to this particular judge.

## The Database

Within the database, you provide the relevant requested material. Crisp, austere presentation is the goal. Avoid extensive dynamic ruminations and obsessive historical detail; cut to the chase.

> Mr. Jones has been a patient of mine for 7 years. I have been treating him for chronic schizophrenia with a regimen of antipsychotic medication and psychotherapy. He has been compliant with his medication and regular in keeping his appointments. His past records and his treatment with me reveal no instances of antisocial behavior or acts of violence.

When a defendant is in treatment, as in this instance, courts are interested in how "good" a patient is—not in a moral sense, but in the sense of following medical directives. It is also obviously meaningful whether he or she is a repeat offender. If there *is* a history of past offenses, list them scrupulously, completely, and objectively; minimizing or whitewashing the facts only hurts your patient ultimately.

A common pitfall for clinicians whose patients have run afoul of the law in some way is to attempt to save the patient by drowning the court in missives filled with exonerating data, character references, promises of good behavior in the future, and so on. This approach will not assist, and may even antagonize, the judge. As mentioned earlier in this chapter, the "Jack Webb approach" ("just the facts, ma'am") is always best. In fact, your objectivity enhances your credibility and your utility to the court and increases the likelihood that your input will be listened to. Having given the facts, leave the court to make its own decisions.

## The Closing

I recommend leaving the door open to further requests, because the information you have provided may miss some point you are unaware of, or the need for further data may emerge from the unwinding of the legal process. Providing specific times when you can be reached is deeply appreciated by busy judges and court clerks:

> I hope this information is useful to you. Please do not hesitate to call me at 555-6666 between 2:00 P.M. and 5:00 P.M., Tuesdays through Thursdays, if I can provide any further information.
>
> Very truly yours,
> (Signature)

## Clearances and Permissions

Psychiatrists are sometimes called on to provide a kind of mental health clearance for a patient. Typical examples include a patient who seeks a driving license, handgun ownership, and employment. In response to such requests, the psychiatrist is, in effect, being asked to predict future performance by the patient—a task that is probably beyond one's clinical powers.

To cope with this problem (extensively addressed elsewhere [1]), I have suggested a double-negative phrasing that avoids seeming to promise success or adequacy while keeping your statements within your clinical capacities:

Based on my examination of March 14, 1995 (or my 2 years of treatment), it is my professional opinion that there are *no* psychiatric *contraindications* to Mr. Jones's obtaining a driver's license. He is at present taking no medications that would be likely to impair his driving skills. (Alternatively, you might state, "He has been cautioned about driving under his present regimen of medications or combining them with alcohol," or "We have reviewed the importance of his taking a course on handgun safety.")

The phrase "no psychiatric contraindications" captures not only the requisite double negative but also the fact that it is only the psychiatric contraindications that can be addressed. Other problems, such as lack of driving skill, are outside your clinical purview. Note that the American Psychiatric Association has published a position statement (titled "Position Statement on Psychiatric Assessment of Driving Ability") on driving matters, stating, in essence, that driving abilities are a matter for registries of motor vehicles and not psychiatric evaluation. Comparably, although psychiatrists understand the risks of handgun availability and violence, we cannot assess someone's competence to use firearms.

## Affidavits

The critical difference between an ordinary letter to a court and an affidavit is that the letter is a simple communication, whereas the affidavit is sworn testimony, just as you might give in the courtroom under oath. This sworn testimony is often conveyed by the phrase just before the signature, "signed under pains and penalties of perjury." Jurisdictions may vary in wording or in the way this matter is approached, but the bottom line is that in a letter, one writes; in an affidavit, one *swears to.* Therefore, be sure of your facts; perjury is not a kidding matter.

As always, when in doubt about what or how to write to a court or agency, having the letter reviewed by a knowledgeable peer or by an attorney will be both useful and reassuring.

# 8

# Specific Roles for the Psychiatrist in Court

The psychiatrist will play a variety of roles in court beyond the general ones outlined in the previous chapters. In this chapter, I focus on some special cases illustrating the difficulties associated with those roles that can be anticipated in court.

## When Your Patient Sues You

Few experiences are as demoralizing as having your patient—in whom you have invested effort, time, skill, patience, and toler-

The author is indebted to Marilyn Berner, J.D., M.S.W., for assistance with the section titled "When Your Patient Sues You."

ance—turn around and sue you for alleged malpractice. Powerful and often unexpected feelings are stirred: outrage at the patient's apparent ingratitude, narcissistic injury, neurotic guilt, grief, depression, panic attacks, imagined shame in your colleagues' eyes, obsessive self-scrutiny to try to find out what you may have done wrong, and full-fledged hatred of the system. Practitioners who have not been sued find it hard to imagine the emotional devastation that can flow from even a baseless suit.

This emotional turmoil may be triggered with the first formal notification that a suit has been brought against you. This notice may be called a demand letter, a claim letter, a legal complaint, or in some sites, a consumer complaint. The language of such letters, although usually standardized and dictated by custom, regulation, or statute, appears to depict you as having the medical competence of a flatworm, the social standing of pond scum, and the moral posture of an ax murderer. You are being put on notice that you will be expected to hand over big bucks for the horrible things you are supposed to have done. At such moments, it may be all but impossible to recall that the language of these letters is, in a sense, as much a matter of theatrics as an attorney's posturing in the courtroom (this point is discussed further later in this chapter).

Note that patients suing their treaters sometimes appear to wish to continue treatment with them. It is a logical paradox but not a clinical one, because litigation may serve a number of complex motivations, not all of which require cessation of treatment. However, the stresses, conflicts, legal pitfalls, and loss of objectivity that come with a malpractice suit preclude resuming or continuing treatment during pendency of the suit (1).

When the time comes to testify as defendant with the patient present in the courtroom, a respectful demeanor and tactful modes of expression should be the rule, despite the emotions you may feel. (Further discussions of the psychology of being sued are listed in the references for this chapter and Appendix 2 at the end of the book.)

A malpractice case as it progresses through the legal system is described in its entirety in the following discussions.

## A Nervous Trot Through the Law

Although my initial plan was to *walk* you through the process of a case, the "gait" in the above heading seemed more suited to the affective context. The following discussions outline the legal system in brief and trot you through the legal stages of a malpractice suit brought against you (for illustrative purposes only, please rest assured). Note also that some of the discussions within this chapter constitute something of a review.

*Statutory law* is the law written in the statutes in law books and also is called *black-letter law.* Thus, if your patient is charged with grand larceny, the definition and penalties for this violation of the statutes are written down and used by the criminal justice system. Statutory law may contain material relevant to civil actions as well, such as the criteria for an expert witness, standards of proof, and definitions of negligence.

*Common law* is the law of specific cases and precedents, built up over time, with occasional changes and emendations. For example, the *Tarasoff* case in California altered the common law by creating a new form of a duty of therapists to protect third parties from a patient's violent acts. Depending on whether cases have transpired on relevant topics, common law may or may not impinge on your participation in a court case. Your lawyer is your guide here.

The criminal justice system is somewhat familiar to most practitioners from television and film, where the various stages are often lingered over in loving detail by the filmmakers to create the drama. From the viewpoint of the psychiatrist whose patient has been caught up in this system, you need only know that a crime involves a violation of a criminal statute and the combination of a wrongful act (*actus reus*) and wrongful intent (*mens rea*). You may be called in at several stages of the procedure to provide mitigating data based on mental illness, aid in sentencing, participate in a probation program, provide postrelease treatment at the end of a sentence, and so on; more formal questions (for example, criminal responsibility) should ordinarily be left to forensic specialists.

The civil system also will involve practitioners, not only as potential defendants in a malpractice suit but also as other types of witnesses discussed in previous chapters in this volume. For psychiatrists, the most relevant aspect of civil litigation is *torts* (civil wrongs), which address wrongs done by one person to another and the mechanisms of compensation for the resultant injury. (See also the discussion in Chapter 2 in this volume. Note that if the injury claimed by a patient of yours is emotional or mental, your psychiatric evaluation and/or testimony may constitute an important part of the proceedings.)

Torts are customarily divided into intentional torts (sins of commission) and unintentional torts (sins of omission). Negligence is a subset of the latter, where the claim is advanced that the defendant (target of the claim) neglected to do something such that he or she fell below the level of ordinary care—what the average person should have foreseen and taken action to prevent. For example, if there is ice on your sidewalk, it is foreseeable that someone may slip and fall, and thus ordinary care means doing something reasonable about it: ice removal, spreading sand, posting a warning sign, etc.

*Professional* negligence is a subset of the former category, an intentional tort, whereby the professional is compared not with the "average person," but with his or her peer group as a reference standard. Hence, the psychiatrist's conduct—action or lack of action—is compared with that of the average reasonable practitioner of psychiatry at the time and under the circumstances (or similar language; it varies somewhat by jurisdiction).

The next focus is the steps along the sometimes years-long *via dolorosa*, which leads to your malpractice suit. The idea has been introduced elsewhere that a malpractice suit results from the malignant synergy of a bad outcome for any reason and bad feelings (1). The mere fact that something bad happened does not alone account for a patient's becoming a plaintiff and bringing litigation. In fact, sad to say, patients seek out lawyers usually after their attempts to set things right with their treaters have been rebuffed.

Another important notion in the law is that of who bears the burden of proof in a given case and what the threshold of proof may be. In criminal cases—in which citizens are innocent until proven guilty—the "state," represented usually by the district attorney, bears the burden of proving guilt beyond a reasonable doubt. Scholars sometimes address this abstraction as a probability of 95% certainty that an individual is guilty.

The plaintiff bears the burden in civil cases, which are usually decided by a standard of "preponderance of the evidence," probabilistically portrayed as "more likely than not" or 51% certainty—a far lower standard than in criminal cases. Certain other types of cases are decided by an intermediate standard of "clear and convincing evidence," sometimes cast as 75% certainty. Examples include termination of parental rights and civil commitment in some jurisdictions.

## Before the Suit Is Filed

In the early stages of the suit, there is some wiggle room (for example, opportunities for negotiation, arbitration, mediation, and repair of the failed alliance). Indeed, the fact that a patient or an attorney is requesting your records out of the blue should be a trigger for your active efforts to contact that patient and open up the dialogue. If you have a hunch that this request might be about litigation, you must also first call your insurer (of course, you should call your insurer when there is any bad outcome, even without litigation looming) to discuss appropriate approaches. On receiving a formal notice of suit, of course, you must call your insurer immediately and let the insurer take it from there. A few points should be made about your early versus later responses that are sometimes overlooked.

First, repair of the therapeutic alliance may well be possible at earlier stages of the game, such as when a patient protests you have treated him or her badly, when your records are requested by a patient (or even by an attorney—be sure to get consultation on this), or when you hear indirectly that a patient is dissatisfied with your care (1). At those early points, contact, discussion, conflict resolution, resumption of treatment, and under some circumstances, careful apology (2) may be not only indicated but also desirable.

However, *after* the lawsuit has been filed, no matter how tempting it may be, *do not* attempt to reach or talk to your patient to find out the problem or even to dissuade him or her somehow from suing you; it is now too late for that. With the actual filing of the lawsuit, such forms of outreach are strictly contraindicated; the situation has become formal and adversarial, and your attorneys should be in charge. All contacts should flow through the attorneys from this point on.

Never forget that a properly expressed apology immediately after a disaster has averted more suits than one can imagine (2) and also that after formal filing, all communication is in the hands of the attorneys.

Note carefully that at this and at almost *every* subsequent stage of the proceedings, an offer to settle may be made. I have even testified in cases in which settlement was reached midtrial—before I even got to the stand. The essence of settlement is that a sum of money is paid to the plaintiff by the defendant and the case goes away—that's all. Almost always, a settlement implies no admission of wrongdoing and thus seems like an excellent way to get on with your life. That, however, is the rub.

When I first entered the forensic field and observed malpractice litigation from the inside, my initial position in advising sued physicians was, "Fight this case to the highest court available; never give up." As my experience grew, I became impressed with the emotional devastation and crushing blow to physicians' morale that a malpractice suit can represent, even a baseless one. My position shifted: I became an advocate of settlement to get cases off the physicians' backs so they could go on with their lives (it is hard to imagine how your life stops when you are being sued).

The newest change regarding litigation involving practitioners is the National Practitioner Data Bank. The obligatory reportage of every settlement, no matter how small, has shifted the balance of decision making somewhat. Some experts argue that it now pays to fight every case because if you win, nothing is reported, and if you lose, you are no worse off than you would be had you settled up front. Although it is true that winning a case keeps your slate clean with the data bank, I suggest that serious consideration still be given to settlement. It is unavoidably true that you will have to explain the suit to every future employer, but this may be worth it in the long run if the suit is predicated on an appropriately minor problem (for example, an unexpected allergic reaction to a medication).

## First Contact

The first news you hear about litigation may be the dreaded letter from the lawyer. There are several forms of this missive. In one version, the attorney simply states that a suit is being brought by Mr. Jones and please notify your insurer. In another, a consumer protection model is followed. Still another outlines every detail of the claim and the allegations supporting it. In any case, when this letter arrives, recall that the time for negotiating is past, and you must now be guided strictly by your attorney to whom all communications from now on must be referred. Failure to follow this rule may jeopardize your case, leave your attorney handicapped, and render your insurer free to pull out of funding your defense—the worst outcome by far.

## The Tribunal or Equivalent

To deal with the malpractice explosion, most jurisdictions set up various forms of screening devices in a well-intentioned effort to screen out trivial or frivolous cases. In some areas, the attorney must obtain a report from a board-certified practitioner that the case has merit on the surface (that is, assuming the claims are true and provable). Other areas use a tribunal, a quasi-judicial hearing in which the case is given a dry run. Tribunals may consist of attorneys and judges or may be a mixed membership of, for example, a physician, a lawyer, and a layperson. Unfortunately, there is no guarantee that the physician on some tribunals will be in the same specialty as the defendant. In practice, in my experience, tribunals actually serve only to screen out ridiculous claims (for example, "That clinician's Trilafon caused me to lose my psychic powers"), but many frivolous ones get through. And even if the tribunal makes a determination against the plaintiff, there are often mechanisms for going ahead with the case anyway, such as by posting a bond for court costs in advance and similar provisions.

## Filing the Suit

The suit is filed in the form a of a complaint against the defendant(s) and becomes, as a legal fact, a matter of public record (that is, the fact that you are being sued, not the details). The defense side may respond by several maneuvers, including answering to the complaint, admitting and denying various parts of the complaint, and making motions to dismiss the suit based on statute of limitations (the suit has been filed too late according to law), failure to state the claim (the allegations do not fit the mold of medical malpractice), absence of duty ("You've got the wrong guy!"), and similar arguments.

## Discovery Phase

The discovery phase is the stage when both sides research the case to determine what the facts are, what the strong and weak points of the case are, and what the experts on both sides think about it. The ultimate purpose of this process is to determine whether a disposition can be reached—drop or settle—or whether a trial is the only possibility. In addition to simply obtaining relevant records, attorneys are permitted to pose certain questions in writing to the other side. The answers to these interrogatories—which your lawyer will work closely with you to answer—are provided under oath and require as scrupulous accuracy of testimony as that in court. Depositions (see Chapter 5 in this volume) are also part of the process. Various maneuvers and countermaneuvers may be initiated by attorneys to determine which questions will not be answered, which depositions will not be taken, and so on. If all settlement efforts fail, a trial will follow.

In almost every case, the attorneys retained by your insurer are top-notch and supportive as well as knowledgeable. I recommend avoiding the temptation, regardless of the stress you feel, to call up your attorney every 4 days to see how the case is progressing. Your attorney will call you when there are any developments worth noting; a lot of "hurry up and wait" is associated with litigation, so do not be surprised if months pass without a word. Meanwhile, *do not* discuss the case with colleagues, because they can be subpoenaed, but *do* feel free to use to their limits your family, therapist, and confidential consultant (someone retained by you for help with your own feelings and stress, whose records are not discoverable, because they do not relate to the patient). Even though their data are not discoverable, the benefit to you is immense.

## Depositions and Other Discovery

The deposition is extensively reviewed in Chapter 5 of this volume and is not repeated here. Refer to that chapter for an in-depth discussion.

## Trial Phase

If all settlement offers fail, the matter eventually may get to trial. Trial conduct and the process are described in Chapters 3 and 6 in this volume. If you prevail at trial, the matter is resolved unless there is an appeal or claim of mistrial; these outcomes prolong the agony. If the plaintiff wins, your insurer negotiates payment of a sum of money, not necessarily what the jury awarded.

## Aftermath

Either outcome—win or lose—at trial must be reported to the National Practitioner Data Bank. Practically, this means that you will be obliged to list and explain this event in future credentialing procedures. This task is burdensome but may not be problematic. In any case, you do your best to go on with your life.

# When Your Patient Sues Someone Else

In today's highly litigious society, it is not uncommon for your patient to be the plaintiff in some litigation against another party. It could be a civil suit regarding motor vehicle accidents, injuries such as slip-and-fall cases, marital conflicts such as divorce, custody and battered spouse claims, or even a malpractice suit against another clinician.

As noted in the discussion of privilege (see Chapter 3 in this volume), if a patient claims emotional injuries, privilege is often waived so that the patient's entire mental health history comes into the legal process. Important implications of this factor may include discussing with the patient whether he or she wishes to open this door, reviewing the notes to anticipate potentially embarrassing material, continuing your supportive role throughout litigation, and resisting the temptation to alter your records, demonize the other side of the case, or draw expert witness–type conclusions about the damages the patient has suffered.

A pitfall for many treaters is to go beyond their own database into the real world in which they were not present as witnesses. The entire body of information from the patient, in other words, could be described as "the patient says, reports, claims, states, alleges," and so on. Although we generally believe what our patients tell us for therapeutic purposes, recall that the courtroom requires a higher standard of proof.

This higher standard of proof is especially true in cases of posttraumatic stress disorder (PTSD), which has appropriately been called a legal minefield (3, 4). One reason that this diagnosis, unlike all other listings in DSM-IV (5), causes such concern is that PTSD posits an actual event—the trauma—as the cause of the presenting symptoms. In other words, presuming a real event and linking causation are elsewhere absent from the deliberately atheoretical DSM-IV. Clinicians must beware of assuming that they know what occurred outside the office, given that all the information they receive is from their patients' (usually uncorroborated) reports. The treaters who overidentify with their patients and who "just know" their patients are reporting accurately actually do their patients a disservice by weakening the treaters' credibility. In objective fact, these treaters *do not* know because they were not there. Treaters who take the attitude that "if my patients said it, it must be true" will become, ironically, their patients' worst enemy in court.

However, as a fact witness—a role you may serve if the patient does claim emotional harms—you are certainly free to describe the signs and symptoms you observed, the diagnoses you made, and the interventions you performed; these are part of your legitimate purview in the case.

# The Patient as Defendant

## Civil Matters

It is quite conceivable that someone may sue your patient for something. In almost every instance, your role will be supportive in helping that patient deal with the stresses of being sued. It is probably essential that you avoid nontherapeutic entanglement in the case; leave that to the lawyers. You often will find that your long-term therapeutic goals and clinical efforts will need to be suspended while you treat the short-term symptomatic responses to the legal process. You may have to accept this moratorium on exploration, because litigation is usually so highly preoccupying that other matters must wait. Discuss this fact candidly with your patient and decide jointly whether to continue in supportive work or to suspend meeting temporarily until the matter is resolved.

## Criminal Matters

If your patient is charged with a crime, the matter may grow slightly more complex. Lawyers may attempt to pervert your knowledge of your patient to aid the legal process, for example, by attempting to fit your patient to the profile of a certain type of offender. Your testimony in this context will be extremely problematic, because it not only may harm your patient but also—because, in the interests of justice, the court may order you to testify—may render irrelevant your patient's permission to testify.

It is probably a good idea to consider delegating various assessments and opinions in the clinical context about your patient to a forensic expert who is removed from the treatment context. This approach is both ethically more sound and more likely to preserve the treatment relationship.

# Other Medicolegal Issues

### Custody Battles

Often called the most malignant legal situation, the custody fight requires comprehensive assessment skills, knowledge of child psychiatry, and expertise in other details outside usual psychiatric practice. The issue of custody battles is beyond the scope of this volume; fortunately, useful literature on this topic exists (6, 7). Experience suggests that custody battle issues should be left to the specialist.

### Involuntary Commitment

For the inpatient psychiatrist, involuntary commitment is a fairly common topic about which the psychiatrist's testimony is required. Concrete data about dangerousness are particularly effective, such as past instances of violence and seclusion and/or restraint episodes on the unit.

### Involuntary Treatment

In some jurisdictions, a psychiatrist may give evidence to courts or quasi-judicial tribunals regarding a patient's competence to consent to or to refuse treatment. Although competence is a *finding* ultimately determined by a court (usually but not always a probate court), a psychiatrist's *opinion* is almost always solicited as to the patient's competence and the indications for the treatment in question. The psychiatrist should keep in mind several important issues about involuntary treatment.

First, note that patients enjoy what all citizens do: a presumption of competence. We are all considered competent unless affirmatively proven otherwise. Mere admission to a psychiatric hospital does not refute this presumption.

A common sign of probable incompetence is denial of a well-established and extensively recorded mental illness. A patient who speaks knowledgeably about the medication but denies the relevance to his or her own condition cannot make reasonable and personal cost-benefit determinations about treatment. Observations by other medical staff are particularly useful and can be presented by the psychiatrist, although some judges will insist on direct testimony from nurses and other staff.

Some jurisdictions use a substituted judgment standard (1) for involuntary treatment. The standard seeks to determine what the now-incompetent patient would want were he or she competent. A history of a patient's continuing to take medication while presumably restored to a competent baseline may be highly relevant and concrete: when competent, the patient *did* seek treatment.

More formal competence determinations, such as competence to make a will, should probably be left to forensic psychiatric specialists.

# References

1. Appelbaum PS, Gutheil TG: Clinical Handbook of Psychiatry and the Law, 2nd Edition. Baltimore, MD, Williams & Wilkins, 1991
2. Gutheil TG: On apologizing to patients. Risk Management Foundation Forum 8:3–4, 1987 (Call the Risk Management Foundation at 617-495-5100.)

3. Simon RI (ed): Posttraumatic Stress Disorder in Litigation. Washington, DC, American Psychiatric Press, 1995

4. Stone AA: Post-traumatic stress disorder and the law: critical review of the new frontier. Bull Am Acad Psychiatry Law 21:23–36, 1993

5. American Psychiatric Association: Diagnostic and Statistical Manual of Mental Disorders, 4th Edition. Washington, DC, American Psychiatric Association, 1994

6. Benedek EP, Schetky DH: Clinical Handbook of Child Psychiatry and the Law. Baltimore, MD, Williams & Wilkins, 1991

7. Gardener RA: Family Evaluation in Child Custody Litigation. Cresskill, NJ, Creative Therapeutics, 1982

# 9

# Epilogue

I hope the information, demystification, and illustrations presented in this book have decreased your fears and concerns about visiting that foreign country, the courtroom. This concise guide should prove handy for quick reference and review if you are faced with the possibility of going to court. And, who knows, your court experiences may even awaken in you a wish to become more involved in the legal system through forensic work. You may be further intrigued by a subspecialty of psychiatry freed from the oppressive constraints of managed care. If so, you may want to read the companion volume, *The Psychiatrist as Expert Witness*. Annual meetings of the American Academy of Psychiatry and the Law (AAPL), the national forensic psychiatric organization, and especially the forensic review course taught there, may further whet your appetite for forensic work, as may the growing number of forensic fellowships available nationally. For more information, call AAPL at 1-800-331-1389.

In addition to this book and the references herein, some other preparatory resources exist. These include consultations with experienced colleagues, visiting the actual courtroom ahead of time, and watching colleagues' testimony either live or on videotape.

The two appendixes at the end of this book may be of further interest to you in your exploration of this anxiety-laden but fascinating area. Appendix 1 is a reprint of a useful article on the issue of whether a treating psychiatrist can serve as an expert witness. Appendix 2 is a list of suggested readings relevant to psychiatry and the law. I hope you find these, too, to be helpful.

# APPENDIX 1

## On Wearing Two Hats: Role Conflict in Serving as Both Psychotherapist and Expert Witness

**Larry H. Strasburger, M.D.,
Thomas G. Gutheil, M.D., and
Archie Brodsky, B.A.**

Should psychotherapists serve as expert witnesses for their patients? Psychotherapists of all disciplines need to confront the potential clinical, legal, and ethical problems involved in combining the roles of treating clinician and forensic evaluator. As clinicians find themselves drawn into proliferating, often ambiguously defined contacts with the legal system, clarity in role definitions becomes crucial.

The authors thank Barbara Long, M.D., and Harold J. Bursztajn, M.D., for their comments and annotations in support of this project and Michael Robbins, M.D., Robert I. Simon, M.D., and Ezra Griffith, M.D., for their review of the manuscript.

# Definitions

The term "therapist" refers to a clinician hired by the patient or the patient's family to provide psychotherapy; therapists treat "patients" or "clients." A "fact witness" testifies as to direct observations that he or she has made; a fact witness does not offer expert opinions or draw conclusions from the reports of others. Thus, a therapist who serves as a fact witness testifies as to observations of the patient during therapy and the immediate conclusions (such as diagnosis and prognosis) drawn from those observations. These conclusions are offered not as an opinion but simply as a report of what the therapist thought, did, and documented during therapy.

An "expert witness" (who may also act as a forensic consultant) is a paid consultant who chooses to become involved in the case and is retained by an attorney, judge, or litigant to provide evaluation and testimony to aid the legal process. Unlike a fact witness, an expert may offer opinions about legal questions. This role typically involves participation in a trial. Forensic experts deal with "examinees" or "evaluees" rather than with patients or clients. They do not attempt to form a doctor-patient relationship with their subjects.

# Common Scenarios

Several common scenarios may prompt a clinician to wear the two hats of treater and expert on behalf of the same person. A patient may have suffered a traumatic incident (such as a criminal assault or an automobile accident) during or before therapy, and litigation may ensue. A patient may become involved in child custody litigation. A referral may come from an attorney ostensibly seeking treatment for a client but actually seeking to document psychiatric damages or obtain favorable testimony in a custody dispute. An individual may be referred by an attorney to a single clinician for both treatment *and* forensic evaluation because the attorney is simply unaware of the incompatibility of these two procedures. Finally, there may be only one practitioner available to provide both psychotherapy and forensic services.

Role conflict may not be immediately apparent to attorneys, patients, or clinicians. Attorneys may believe that by enlisting the treating clinician as a forensic expert, they are making efficient use of the most knowledgeable source of information. After all, who is closer to the patient than his or her own therapist? Moreover, current ethical opinions of the American Medical Association state, "If a patient who has a legal claim requests a physician's assistance, the physician should furnish medical evidence" (1). The attorney may also want to save money: "Why bring in a new person, who probably charges even higher fees than the treating psychotherapist, for an evaluation the therapist can easily perform?" The patient, too, may object to a separate forensic evaluation: "Why must I repeat a painful story, and to someone I don't already know and trust?" The therapist, in the throes of countertransference (2) as well as anxious to spare the patient needless suffering, may readily endorse this reasoning. Clinicians who lack forensic training may think it natural to extend the mission of supporting the patient in therapy to advocating for the patient in court.

## The Core Conflicts

It is prudent for clinicians to resist both the external pressures emanating from the attorney or patient or both and the internal pressures from the therapist's felt allegiance to the patient. The legal process is directed toward the resolution of disputes; psychotherapy pursues the medical goal of healing. Although these purposes need not always be antithetical and may even be congruent, the processes themselves typically create an irreconcilable role conflict.

In essence, treatment in psychotherapy is brought about through an empathic relationship that has no place in, and is unlikely to survive, the questioning and public reporting of a forensic evaluation. To assume either role in a particular case is to compromise one's capacity to fulfill the other. This role conflict, analyzed in detail later in this article, manifests itself in different conceptions of truth and causation, different forms of alliance, different types of assessment, and different ethical guidelines (3). Therefore, although circumstances may make the assumption of the dual role necessary and/or unavoidable, the problems that surround this practice argue for its avoidance whenever possible.

Writing in 1984, Miller (4) noted that concern about this form of dual relationship "has seldom appeared in the literature" (p. 826). Even now, it is remarkable how little critical attention this major ethical issue has received, even in articles and texts purporting to offer comprehensive expositions of the ethics of forensic practice (5). A brief review of the professional literature shows the need for a more definitive analysis.

## Historical Overview—
## A Slowly Emerging Issue

Role conflict has come to preoccupy the psychotherapeutic professions as the legal, economic, and social ramifications of their work have multiplied. An early expression of this concern was Stanton and Schwartz's exploration of the therapist-versus-administrator dilemma (6). In the 1970s the term "double agent," both in psychotherapy (7) and in medicine (8), came to signify the clinician's joint responsibilities to the patient and the state.

These early critiques, however, generally neglected to ask whether the evaluee's treating therapist is the right person to perform a forensic evaluation. Even in the early forensic psychiatric literature, clear linguistic distinctions between a forensic and a clinical examination (9) and between a forensic evaluee and a patient (10) were not always maintained. As late as 1987, a major textbook on forensic evaluation (11) did not directly address the treater-as-expert question.

An emerging emphasis on separating the clinical and legal roles was articulated in Stone's 1983 advice to therapists who learn that a patient may have been sexually abused by another therapist (12). Stone recommended that the therapist discharge the ethical responsibilities of confidentiality and neutrality by engaging a consultant to pursue legal and administrative remedies on the patient's (and the public's) behalf. The following year, Halleck made the most explicit mention to date of the treater/expert role conflict in the literature on the double agent (13). Since then, a few clear warnings about such role conflict have appeared in the literature of forensic psychiatry (14, 15) and forensic psychology (16), but these have been oases in a desert.

## Ethics Codes

The problematic treater/expert relationship differs from the dual relationships commonly proscribed in ethics codes of professional organizations (17) in that it represents a conflict between two professional roles rather than between a professional and a nonprofessional one. This particular role conflict is addressed most directly by the American Academy of Psychiatry and the Law in its *Ethical Guidelines for the Practice of Forensic Psychiatry*:

> A treating psychiatrist should generally avoid agreeing to be an expert witness or to perform an evaluation of his patient for legal purposes because a forensic evaluation usually requires that other people be interviewed and testimony may adversely affect the therapeutic relationship (18).

Sound as they are, these guidelines not only lack detailed elaboration, but are unenforceable, since the American Academy of Psychiatry and the Law refers ethics complaints to APA, which has not adopted the Academy's ethical guidelines. APA has, however, issued a comparable position statement with respect to employment-related psychiatric examinations (19).

For psychologists, the ethical boundary is less sharply drawn. The American Psychological Association's code of ethics (20) allows psychologists to serve simultaneously as consultant or expert and as fact witness in the same case, provided that they "clarify role expectations" (p. 1610). Guidelines developed specifically for forensic psychologists by the American Psychology-Law Society and Division 41 of the American Psychological Association (21) address the "potential conflicts of interest in dual relationships with parties to a legal proceeding" (p. 659). These guidelines, however, allow broader latitude than those of the American Academy of Psychiatry and the Law.

## Surveys of Forensic Psychiatrists

Surveys of forensic psychiatrists' ethical concerns reveal a surprising lack of consensus on the treater/expert role conflict. In a 1986 survey of forensic psychiatrists who belonged to the American Academy of Forensic Sciences, two-thirds considered "conflicting loyalties" a significant ethical issue, yet only three of 51 respondents specifically mentioned the treater/evaluator role conflict (22). In 1989, with the ethical guidelines of the American Academy of Psychiatry and the Law recently in place, members of both the American Academy of Forensic Sciences and the American Academy of Psychiatry and the Law rated the treater/expert scenario least significant among 28 potential ethical problems listed (23). (Only 14.5% of the members of the American Academy of Forensic Sciences perceived this situation to represent an ethical problem, while 71.0% did not.)

In 1991, among 12 controversial ethical guidelines proposed for consideration, members of the American Academy of Psychiatry and the Law gave least support to extending the Academy's warning against performing forensic evaluations on current patients to include former patients as well (24). The authors of the survey attributed this opposition, as well as continuing disagreement even about the impropriety of evaluating current patients, to a "recognition of the dual treater-evaluator role sometimes being both necessary and appropriate" (p. 245). Thus, during the past decade, any increased scrutiny of this dual role has confronted the reasoning that "multiple agency and a balancing of values have become a necessary part of all current psychiatric practice, not only for forensic psychiatry" (p. 246).

## Contexts and Complications

The resistance of highly trained specialists to such an ethical principle becomes understandable when set against the changing land-
scape of psychotherapy. Limited reimbursements are making
extended psychodynamic exploration a luxury. Moreover, with
many patients' problems being seen as manifestations of extrapsy-
chic (environmental, institutional, economic, legal, or political)
conditions, the therapist is becoming a social worker, mobilizing
resources on the patient's behalf; a gatekeeper, unlocking the
doors of managed care; a detective, obtaining useful information;
or an agent of social control, protecting others from the patient.
The therapist, thus placed in an advocate's or case manager's role,
is expected to influence external outcomes rather than simply accompany the patient on an inner exploration.

Mental health services today are commonly delivered in public
institutions (such as state hospitals and prisons) where therapists
are accountable to society as well as to the patient. In these settings confidentiality may be breached from the outset, and therapy
often has a built-in forensic component. Even private psychotherapy takes on a forensic dimension in the case of reportable offenses or threats to third parties. To some degree, then, the
treater/expert role conflict has become incorporated into the
therapist's job description. "Pure," disinterested psychotherapy is
compromised as legal, economic, and social responsibilities multi-
ply and fewer clinicians really practice independently. More and
more, the therapist is working for institutions, corporations, and
society.

Given these conditions, rigorous separation of the treater and
evaluator roles in public practice has been called unworkable and
even inadvisable (25). Nonetheless, a strong reaffirmation of role
clarity is still called for, especially in light of an epidemic of aggres-
sive legal advocacy by therapists. The proliferation of cases of "recovered memory," for instance, with their dubious methodologies
and controversial outcomes, shows that some therapists are losing
sight of the essential distinction between subjective experience

and historical reconstruction (26). These therapists, perhaps driven by unexamined countertransference (2), step out of role when they urge their patients to take to court issues that might better be resolved in therapy.

For didactic clarity, the following discussion is cast in the language of traditional psychotherapy. Nonetheless, it applies to many forms of psychiatric and psychological treatment, including psychopharmacological, behavioral, and cognitive therapies. Since questions of trust, rapport, and confidentiality enter into all clinical treatment, the evaluator's role of gathering and reporting information from multiple sources external to the dyad is always in conflict with the treater's role.

# Truth and Causation

Clinical and forensic undertakings are dissimilar in that they are directed at different (although overlapping) realities, which they seek to understand in correspondingly different ways.

## Psychic Reality Versus Objective Reality

The process of psychotherapy is a search for meaning more than for facts. In other words, it may be conceived of more as a search for narrative truth (a term now in common use) than for historical truth (27). Whereas the forensic examiner is skeptical, questioning even plausible assertions for purposes of evaluation (28), the therapist may be deliberately credulous, provisionally "believing" even implausible assertions for therapeutic purposes. The therapist accepts the patient's narrative as representing an inner, personal reality, albeit colored by biases and misperceptions. This narrative is not expected to be a veridical history; rather, the therapist strives to see the world "through the patient's eyes." Personal mythologies are reviewed, constructed, and remodeled as an individual reflects on himself or herself and his or her functioning.

Although the therapist withholds judgment and does not rush

to reach (let alone impose) a conclusion, the ultimate goal is to guide the patient to a more objective understanding. Nonetheless, the achievement of insight, one of the principal goals of psychotherapy, is not a fact-finding mission and cannot be reliably audited by an external source. What emerges with insight often cannot be objectively corroborated, confirmed, or validated so as to meet legal standards of proof.

One possible consequence of the clinician's tactical suspension of disbelief in the patient's subjective reality is that a plaintiff's psychotherapist may fail to diagnose malingering (29). If the patient's agenda, conscious or unconscious or both, includes building a record for future court testimony, a psychotherapeutic goal will not be achieved, whether or not the therapist eventually testifies. Distortions of emphasis and a withholding of information, affect, and associations will likely compromise both the therapy and the testimony. Therefore, in cases that may have legal ramifications, the limits of the therapist's role with respect to forensic evaluations and court testimony should be made clear as part of the treatment contract. Of course, the therapist cannot always anticipate the litigable issues that may emerge in therapy or assume that an initial disclaimer will dispose of the patient's unconscious agendas.

## Descriptive Versus Dynamic Approach

Whereas the treating clinician looks out from within, the forensic expert, who must adhere to an ethical standard of objectivity (18), looks in from outside. Thus, whereas the treater might appropriately take a psychodynamic perspective, with its emphasis on conflict and the role of the unconscious, the forensic evaluator's view is more likely to be a descriptive one. The objective/descriptive approach to psychiatry, with its emphasis on classification and reliable diagnosis, tends to be favored by forensic practitioners because the law is interested in categorization. Diagnosis A may be compensable or potentially exculpatory, while diagnosis B may not be.

This is not to say that the stereotypical forensic psychiatrist, who reconstructs an individual's inner world (if at all) only from tangible (e.g., crime scene) evidence, is truly representative of this specialty. It may well be that forensic psychiatry is best practiced by those who can immerse themselves in the evaluee's inner world and then exit that world with useful observations and testable hypotheses in a search for corroboration or lack of corroboration. For the most part, however, the law sees human beings as operating consciously, rationally, and deliberately (30). Although it allows for mental state defenses and gives selective attention to particular dynamic mechanisms, such as transference in sexual misconduct litigation (31), the law has little interest in the unconscious.

On the other side of the coin, although a therapist may have a high degree of confidence in a patient's clinical diagnosis, this determination is not to be confused with the forensic evaluator's effort to document an accurate historical reconstruction. A therapist must tolerate ambiguity to such a degree as to be often unable to answer a legal question with the "reasonable degree of medical certainty" (32) required of an expert opinion. To say, "I am reasonably certain that this person is presenting with posttraumatic stress disorder," is not to say, "It is my opinion, to a reasonable degree of medical certainty, that the trauma was caused by the sexual abuse she says she suffered at her father's hands." Equating these two statements is a damaging mistake that clinicians unfamiliar with the courts often make when they move into the legal arena.

# The Nature of the Alliance

The clinical and forensic situations differ with respect to the nature and purpose of the relationships formed within them. Involvement in litigation inevitably affects the empathy, neutrality, and anonymity of the clinician.

## Psychological Versus Social Purpose

Like the psychotherapist and patient, the forensic evaluator and evaluee jointly undertake a task. But the two tasks are not the same. In treatment, the purpose of the alliance is the psychological one of benefiting the patient by promoting healing and enlarging the sphere of personal awareness, responsibility, choice, and self-care. In the forensic context the purpose is the social one of benefiting society by promoting fair dispute resolution through the adversarial legal system. At its best, the forensic psychiatric evaluation has been characterized as sharing some qualities of a working alliance but only for the limited purpose of conducting the evaluation (28).

Because amelioration through civil law usually takes the form of financial compensation, the contrast between the two alliances is, in one sense, that of making whole psychologically versus making whole economically. These separate restitutions only sometimes overlap. The respective outcomes may also be thought of as insight versus justice, as changing primarily the internal world rather than the external world. In the course of a therapeutic alliance the patient must often accept personal responsibility as a condition of change. This contrasts strongly with the plaintiff's quest to assign responsibility to others in order to achieve recompense, cost sharing, or equity—as well as vindication. In therapy, the patient frequently must learn to understand and forgive; these considerations are largely irrelevant to the forensic evaluee and antithetical to the retributive thrust of litigation.

In building a treatment alliance the psychotherapist attempts to ally with that part of the patient that seeks to change, to give up psychopathological symptoms, and to resume or develop healthy adaptations (33). The perspective is future oriented; troubles should be ameliorated for a better, happier life. Entitlements may have to be discarded so that one can cope with everyday existence. One must accept that life is hard and often unjust and assume responsibility for one's role.

The forensic evaluator, on the other hand, may be allied with (or else opposed to) that part of the evaluee which seeks concrete redress for injury, exculpation from responsibility, or avoidance of responsibility through a finding of incompetence. The evaluator's approach may emphasize psychopathology, in contrast to the normalizing approach of the psychotherapist. The attention paid to a psychopathological slice of past life, without any hope-giving search for renewal and remediation, may foster a depressive rather than an encouraging outlook.

People often bring legal action in the belief that it will be therapeutic and empowering. Sometimes it is, but it can also be traumatic. Moreover, the sense of entitlement fostered by an unremitting quest for justice tends to harden characterological defenses, thereby making constructive change more elusive. In such cases, litigation may be said to bring about a developmental arrest or regression antithetical to therapeutic growth. Given such risks, the proper role of a treating therapist is not to encourage a lawsuit or to be the patient's legal advocate. Rather, it is to assist the patient in deciding whether or not to bring suit and to provide support in going through the legal process, if that be the decision. The therapist ought to stand at the same distance from the lawsuit as from any other significant event in the patient's life.

## Empathy

Empathy, when used as a therapeutic technique, enables the patient to feel understood and facilitates the achievement of insight. Contrary to stereotype, empathy is not necessarily absent from the forensic evaluation, since a skilled evaluator creates an atmosphere in which the evaluee feels free to speak within the limits set by the absence of confidentiality (28). However, even the legitimate use of empathy can lead to a quasi-therapeutic interaction that ultimately leaves the evaluee feeling betrayed by the evaluator's report (34).

The clinician's habit of empathic identification, if not balanced by objectivity, can bias a forensic evaluation even in the absence of a treating relationship. Stone (35) argues, therefore, that forensic evaluators must be prepared to withdraw from the forensic role when a forensic evaluation turns into a therapeutic encounter. How much greater, then, the likelihood of bias in the case of a treating therapist, whose mission of promoting patient welfare calls for deliberate identification (at the risk of overidentification) with the patient.

## Neutrality

Therapeutic neutrality (36)—that posture of helping the patient listen to himself or herself without critical judgment, and fostering self-knowledge through the emergence of hidden feelings and attitudes—is undermined when the clinician acts as a forensic consultant to the patient or attorney; judgmental assessments are inevitable in that role, and serious real-world consequences may turn on every utterance of the patient. The crucial therapeutic posture of expectant listener, to whom anything may be said without consequence or penalty, is compromised. Free access to the patient's inner world is impeded as each disclosure is weighed, not just against "What will she [or he] think of me?" but also "How will what I say affect the outcome of my case?" Neutrality vanishes as the therapist assumes the consultant's role of advocacy for an opinion supporting the patient's cause (37), a role assumed in the U.S. Supreme Court's *Ake* decision (38). Both patient's and therapist's rescue fantasies are activated, with their potential for idealization of the therapist and regression and infantilization of the patient. Patient autonomy and responsibility correspondingly diminish.

## Anonymity

The anonymity of the psychotherapist, which aids in the development and interpretation of transference (39) and the mobilization of clinically useful projections onto the therapist, is clearly compromised by the legal process. Such anonymity, which may be a key to the residual attitudes of the patient's relationships with important figures in his or her past, is contaminated when the therapist steps out of the transference relationship and into the patient's present, external world. The patient who sees his or her therapist on the witness stand may have strong reactions, not only to the testimony itself, but to whatever is exposed about the clinician's professional background, character, or personal history. Problems also arise if the patient sees the therapist embarrassed by a vigorous and effective cross-examination. Will confidence and trust not be diminished by fears of the therapist's vulnerability?

# Assessments

Further incompatibilities between the roles of treater and expert become apparent when we consider how each obtains, evaluates, and interprets information. A clinical assessment is not the same as a forensic assessment.

## Evidence Gathering and the Use of Collateral Sources

Therapeutic assessments tend to rely much less on collateral sources of information than do forensic evaluations. While spouses and other family members may be interviewed (with the patient's permission) as part of a clinical assessment—particularly for hospitalized or substance-abusing patients—a forensic evaluation routinely requires meticulous examination of multiple sources of information, such as medical, insurance, school, and occupational records, as well as interviews with family members, co-workers, employers, friends, police officers, and eyewitnesses. Such far-ranging scrutiny by a psychotherapist, especially in outpatient treatment, would be highly unusual. Indeed, were a therapist to seek external "truth" so diligently, the patient might well exclaim, "Doctor, don't you believe me?"

In practice, forensic assessments may also include observing the evaluee in the home, the workplace, the courtroom, and other non-clinical settings. Except in some types of couple or family therapy, comparable behavior by a psychotherapist would likely be perceived by the patient as highly intrusive (and hence destructive of confidence and trust) or as a therapeutic boundary violation (40).

## Interview Strategies

Psychotherapists and forensic psychiatrists approach their patients/evaluees with divergent interviewing strategies. The forensic psychiatrist begins with an explicit legal question to be answered by marshalling relevant psychiatric data (41). For the psychotherapist this external question would be a distraction from the patient's inner world and therapeutic goals. Moreover, the direct probing necessary for forensic evaluation is inconsistent with the "evenly hovering attention" (42, pp. 111–112) of the dynamic psychiatrist. Using an open-ended approach, the psychotherapist starts with the problem as perceived by the patient and proceeds to collect an associative anamnesis (43) intended to yield a dynamic understanding of the issues. The language of the therapist deliberately emulates that of the patient, who is encouraged to tell his or her own story in his or her own way.

In contrast, the forensic evaluator's gaining informed consent to the interview opens with a defining statement of purpose. While the forensic examiner's initial inquiries may be phrased open-endedly to encourage the interviewee's participation, the questioning becomes increasingly structured in keeping with implicit legal standards, if not the actual statutory issue and vocabulary. (In some jurisdictions, such as New York, the evaluee is permitted to have a lawyer present, giving the interview the cast of a legal deposition rather than a clinical interview.) If such an examination is undertaken by the treating psychotherapist, it may well be experienced by the patient as a failure of empathy.

## Psychological Defenses

Psychotherapy, the "talking cure," requires that thoughts and feelings be put into words in order to effect change. While enactments of various past and present conflicts inevitably occur and, indeed, are often instructive when they can be explored, verbal communication is the mode of choice. In any psychotherapy, resistances and defenses may impede the work. Litigation tends to enhance these defensive maneuvers: it may provide a defense against experiencing affect or a distraction from considering meaningful aspects of the past. Thus, a therapist who is drawn into a patient's litigation is participating in an enactment or acting out.

## Time

Time limitations also differentiate forensic from treatment evaluations, except for certain deliberately short-term therapeutic techniques. A sense of urgency and a need to move toward closure, while characteristic of managed care settings, are not inherent to traditional psychotherapy. Except in an emergency, the treating psychiatrist usually has some leeway to wait for material to emerge in its own time or to wait to intervene until the moment is right. The intrinsic schedule is that of the patient, not that of the court. The forensic specialist usually does not have this luxury. "Having one's day in court" requires respect for deadlines and inevitably leads to temporal closure, whether or not clinical end points have been reached.

## Ethical Guidelines

Problems occur when the ethic of healing (doing "individual good") collides with the ethic of objectively serving the legal system (doing "social good"). The following are some of the ethical dilemmas that arise when one attempts to serve one client in two arenas.

### "First, Do No Harm"

The ethical dictum of *primum non nocere,* by which treating physicians are bound, does not apply directly in the courtroom (44). An evaluee may suffer substantial harm from a forensic expert's testimony, not only through lost self-esteem, financial loss, or deprivation of liberty, but even through loss of life in capital sentencing. Moreover, the damage done by inadequate or ineffective testimony resulting from a therapist's incomplete understanding of the legal system may be financially as well as emotionally costly (45). Even when the testifying expert is a qualified forensic specialist, the experience of hearing one's intimate life revealed and analyzed in court may be exceedingly traumatic (46).

Mossman (47) opines that honest forensic evaluations and testimony, even when they do immediate harm to individuals, confer long-range benefits on all concerned (including those adversely affected) by upholding the fairness of the justice system. Nonetheless, that way of doing good is not part of the *treating* physician's role. A person who suffers harm from adverse or painful testimony should not suffer the additional pain of having that testimony emerge from a doctor-patient relationship.

## Reimbursement

Another ethical issue arises when the psychotherapist goes to court. If a prognosis is offered that a patient will require long-term treatment, the therapist, as treater, stands to benefit directly from this statement (29). This financial stake in the outcome may destroy the credibility of the therapist's testimony. It places the therapist in the position of testifying for a built-in contingency fee, which is unethical for forensic psychiatrists (18) and forensic psychologists (21)—and, by extension, for treaters who testify.

## Agency

Clear disclosure of whose "agent" one serves as—i.e., whom one is working for—is required in both the clinical and forensic arenas. Barring an emergency, including danger to others or "public peril," a therapist works only for the patient. Such an "agency statement" is usually implicit in a contract between psychiatrist and patient for individual psychotherapy (33). In the forensic context, however, the combined therapist/expert witness must serve two masters, the patient/examinee and the law. When the therapist thus blurs his or her role, the patient's claim to sole allegiance is compromised.

The biasing effect of agency on forensic evaluations, a matter of concern to forensic specialists (48), is called forensic identification—a process by which evaluators unintentionally adopt the viewpoint of the attorneys who have retained them (49). If agency biases forensic opinion, agency conflict, or double agency, must influence both the evaluator (therapist) and evaluee (patient).

## Confidentiality

The question of confidentiality goes hand in hand with that of agency. Who is listening? What will be revealed and where? The privacy of the consulting room, protected by law, is essential to frank communication during which a patient suspends self-judgment. In its *Jaffee v. Redmond* decision in 1996 (50), the U.S. Supreme Court gave unequivocal protection to the confidentiality of the psychotherapeutic relationship. Given the Court's reaffirmation of the primacy of therapeutic confidentiality, over and above other vital interests of society, clinicians would be unwise to compromise this right by carelessly crossing the boundary into the forensic arena.

A patient who puts his or her mental condition at legal issue and thereby waives privilege loses that privacy. Although the patient may consent to breaching privacy for the purpose of litigation, the prior confidential relationship may be incapable of being restored after the litigation is over. Moreover, the patient's consent to reveal treatment records may not constitute informed consent to full disclosure in court to family members, the press, or curious bystanders (46). A warning that the adversarial discovery process may reveal closely held personal details may not address the full extent of the exposure that occurs and its emotional consequences.

These hazards of litigation are present whether or not the therapist actually testifies. If the therapist agrees to act as a forensic evaluator, the hazards intensify. While a treating therapist may sometimes successfully appeal to exclude intimate material because of its irrelevance, the forensic evaluator is less likely to be able to withhold anything learned in the course of an evaluation.

## Risks for the Clinician
## Who Acts in a Dual Role

At a time when forensic experts have been held liable for negligence in evaluation (51), the therapist who attempts to combine the roles of treating clinician and forensic evaluator embarks on especially treacherous waters. Even a clinician who testifies as a fact witness may find this seemingly unambiguous role compromised (50). In court, the fact witness may face pressure to give an expert opinion without receiving an expert witness's fee (52). Worse, a therapist whose factual testimony displeases the patient may later be charged with negligence for having failed to carry out the investigatory tasks of a forensic expert (53).

These problems are best avoided by offering the patient's treatment records in lieu of testimony. The clinician who does testify as a fact witness should rigorously maintain role boundaries by declining to perform the functions of an expert witness, such as reviewing the reports or depositions of other witnesses. A therapist who is asked to give expert testimony about a patient can respond to an attorney's request, a subpoena, or (at last resort) courtroom questioning with a disclaimer such as this: "Having observed the patient only from the vantage point of a treating clinician, I have no objective basis for rendering an expert opinion, with a reasonable degree of medical certainty, on a legal as opposed to a clinical question."

## Caveats

1. *Ruling out this form of dual relationship is not meant to limit the expert role to a small group of specialists.* Any professional can serve as an expert witness within the limits of his or her expertise. A psychiatrist without specialized credentials in forensic psychiatry can still perform evaluations and testify as an expert in psychiatry.

2. *Separating the roles of treater and expert implies no denigration of clinical expertise.* "Expert witness" is a legal term that describes the particular role a person plays in the legal process. To insist that the role of an expert witness is incompatible with that of a treating clinician is not to imply that clinicians are any less expert in their own realm.

3. *Treating clinicians do have legitimate roles in legal proceedings.* Treating clinicians properly participate in certain legal determinations as part of their clinical responsibilities. For example, the assessment of competence to give informed consent

to treatment is inherently part of the clinical interchange. Similarly, the clinician who petitions a court for involuntary commitment of a patient usually testifies as a fact witness—an involved party, a partisan for safety and patient health—about his or her observations of the patient during therapy. There is, however, an inherent ambiguity in this role in that legal conclusions are being reached on the basis of the testimony. Although the clinician's temporary assumption of an oppositional role in court for the patient's benefit may strain the therapeutic alliance, inpatient treatment can restore the patient's insight, so that the patient comes to understand why hospitalization was necessary and the treatment alliance can resume.

4. *Sometimes the dual role* is *unavoidable.* Institutional policies increasingly force clinicians to wear two hats with the same patient. Similarly, in commitment hearings and disability determinations the clinician may be drawn into a quasi-expert role. Geography can also be a limiting factor; in a small town or rural area there may be only one practitioner available with the requisite credentials to perform a forensic evaluation (54). Even in less than ideal circumstances, however, one should be vigilant to avoid compromising one's role, especially through unnecessary breaches of confidentiality (50).

## Conclusions

The psychotherapist's wish to help the patient too often carries over into more direct, active forms of "helping" that (however well-motivated) are contrary to the therapeutic mission. In particular, a therapist's venturing into forensic terrain may be understood as a boundary violation that can compromise therapy as surely and as fatally as other, more patently unethical transgressions. For the numerous reasons detailed previously, such dual agency is unsound and potentially damaging both to the evaluee/patient and to the evaluator/clinician. As the psychotherapist's role boundaries widen, there is a proportional increase in the intensity of ethical conflict and legal liability. Notwithstanding the growing pressures from the complex clinical/legal marketplace to perform simultaneously in multiple roles, two heads are better than one only if they really are two distinct heads, each wearing its own hat.

# References

1. American Medical Association, Council on Ethical and Judicial Affairs: Code of Medical Ethics: Current Opinions With Annotations. Chicago, AMA, 1994, p 138
2. Long BL: Psychiatric diagnoses in sexual harassment cases. Bull Am Acad Psychiatry Law 1994; 22:195–203
3. Hundert EM: Competing medical and legal ethical values: balancing problems of the forensic psychiatrist, in Ethical Practice in Psychiatry and the Law. Edited by Rosner R, Weinstock R. New York, Plenum, 1990, pp 53–72
4. Miller RD: The treating psychiatrist as forensic evaluator. J Forensic Sci 1984; 29:825–830
5. Golding SL: Mental health professionals and the courts: the ethics of expertise. Int J Law Psychiatry 1990; 13:281–307
6. Stanton A, Schwartz M: The Mental Hospital. New York, Basic Books, 1954
7. Gaylin W: In the Service of the State: The Psychiatrist as Double Agent: Hastings Center Report Special Supplement. New York, Institute of Society, Ethics and Life Sciences, 1978
8. Lomas HD, Berman JD: Diagnosing for administrative purposes: some ethical problems. Soc Sci Med 1983; 17:241–244
9. Watson AS: On the preparation and use of psychiatric expert testimony: some suggestions in an ongoing controversy. Bull Am Acad Psychiatry Law 1978; 6:226–246
10. Rappeport JR: Differences between forensic and general psychiatry. Am J Psychiatry 1982; 139:331–334
11. Melton GB, Petrila J, Poythress NG, Slobogin C: Psychological Evaluations for the Courts. New York, Guilford Press, 1987
12. Stone AA: Sexual misconduct by psychiatrists: the ethical and clinical dilemma of confidentiality. Am J Psychiatry 1983; 140:195–197
13. Halleck SL: The ethical dilemmas of forensic psychiatry: a utilitarian approach. Bull Am Acad Psychiatry Law 1984; 12:279–288

14. Group for the Advancement of Psychiatry, Committee on Psychiatry and Law: The Mental Health Professional and the Legal System: Report 131. New York, Brunner/Mazel, 1991

15. Epstein RS: Keeping Boundaries: Maintaining Safety and Integrity in the Psychotherapeutic Process. Washington, DC, American Psychiatric Press, 1994

16. Shapiro DL: Forensic Psychological Assessment: An Integrative Approach. Boston, Allyn & Bacon, 1991

17. Rinella VJ, Gerstein AI: The development of dual relationships: power and professional responsibility. Int J Law Psychiatry 1994; 17: 225–237

18. American Academy of Psychiatry and the Law: Ethical Guidelines for the Practice of Forensic Psychiatry. Bloomfield, Conn, AAPL, 1991

19. American Psychiatric Association: Position statement on employment-related psychiatric examinations. Am J Psychiatry 1985; 142:416

20. American Psychological Association: Ethical principles of psychologists and code of conduct. Am Psychol 1992; 47:1597–1611

21. Committee on Ethical Guidelines for Forensic Psychologists: Specialty guidelines for forensic psychologists. Law and Human Behavior 1991; 15:655–665

22. Weinstock R: Ethical concerns expressed by forensic psychiatrists. J Forensic Sci 1986; 31:596–602

23. Weinstock R: Perceptions of ethical problems by forensic psychiatrists. Bull Am Acad Psychiatry Law 1989; 17:189–202

24. Weinstock R, Leong GG, Silva JA: Opinions by AAPL forensic psychiatrists on controversial ethical guidelines: a survey. Bull Am Acad Psychiatry Law 1991; 19:237–248

25. Miller RD: Ethical issues involved in the dual role of treater and evaluator, in Ethical Practice in Psychiatry and the Law. Edited by Rosner R, Weinstock R. New York, Plenum, 1990, pp 129–150

26. Gutheil TG: True or false memories of sexual abuse? a forensic psychiatric view. Psychiatr Annals 1993; 23:527–531

27. Spence DP: Narrative Truth and Historical Truth: Meaning and Interpretation in Psychoanalysis. New York, WW Norton, 1982

28. Bursztajn HJ, Scherr AE, Brodsky A: The rebirth of forensic psychiatry in light of recent historical trends in criminal responsibility. Psychiatr Clin North Am 1994; 17:611–635

29. Simon RI: Toward the development of guidelines in the forensic psychiatric examination of posttraumatic stress disorder claimants, in Posttraumatic Stress Disorder in Litigation: Guidelines for Forensic Assessment. Edited by Simon RI. Washington, DC, American Psychiatric Press, 1995, pp 31–84

30. Morse SJ: Brain and blame. Georgetown Law J 1996; 84:527–549

31. Gutheil TG: Some ironies in psychiatric sexual misconduct litigation: editorial and critique. Newsletter of the Am Acad Psychiatry and Law 1992; 17:56–59

32. Rappeport JR: Reasonable medical certainty. Bull Am Acad Psychiatry Law 1985; 13:5–16

33. Gutheil TG, Havens LL: The therapeutic alliance: contemporary meanings and confusions. Int Rev Psychoanal 1979; 6:467–481

34. Shuman DW: The use of empathy in forensic examinations. Ethics & Behavior 1993; 3:289–302

35. Stone AA: Revisiting the parable: truth without consequences. Int J Law Psychiatry 1994; 17:79–97

36. Hoffer A: Toward a definition of psychoanalytic neutrality. J Am Psychoanal Assoc 1985; 33:771–795

37. Diamond BL: The fallacy of the impartial expert. Arch Criminal Psychodynamics 1959; 3:221–236

38. Ake v Oklahoma, 105 S Ct 1087 (1985)

39. Freud S: Observations on transference-love: further recommendations on the technique of psycho-analysis, III (1915 [1914]), in Complete Psychological Works, standard ed, vol 12. London, Hogarth Press, 1958, pp 157–173

40. Gutheil TG, Gabbard GO: The concept of boundaries in clinical practice: theoretical and risk-management dimensions. Am J Psychiatry 1993; 150:188–196

41. Rosner R: A conceptual framework for forensic psychiatry, in Principles and Practice of Forensic Psychiatry. Edited by Rosner R. New York, Chapman & Hall, 1994, pp 3–6

42. Freud S: Recommendations to physicians practising psycho-analysis (1912), in Complete Psychological Works, standard ed, vol 12. London, Hogarth Press, 1958, pp 109–120

43. Deutsch F, Murphy WF: The Clinical Interview, vol I: Diagnosis: A Method of Teaching Associative Exploration. New York, International Universities Press, 1955

44. Appelbaum PS: The parable of the forensic psychiatrist: ethics and the problem of doing harm. Int J Law Psychiatry 1990; 13:249–259

45. Carmichael v Carmichael, Washington, DC, Court of Appeals Number 89-1524

46. Strasburger LH: "Crudely, without any finesse": the defendant hears his psychiatric evaluation. Bull Am Acad Psychiatry Law 1987; 15: 229–233

47. Mossman D: Is expert psychiatric testimony fundamentally immoral? Int J Law Psychiatry 1994; 17:347–368

48. Rogers R: Ethical dilemmas in forensic evaluations. Behavioral Science and Law 1987; 5:149–160

49. Zusman J, Simon J: Differences in repeated psychiatric examinations of litigants to a lawsuit. Am J Psychiatry 1983; 140:1300–1304

50. Jaffee v Redmond et al, 1996 WL 315841 (US)

51. Weinstock R, Garrick T: Is liability possible for forensic psychiatrists? Bull Am Acad Psychiatry Law 1995; 23:183–193

52. Brun v Bailey, Number CO11911, Court of Appeal of California, Third Appellate District. 27 Cal App 4th 641; 1994 Cal App LEXUS 833; 32 Cal Rptr 2d 624

53. Althaus v Cohen and WPIC, Federal Civil Action Number 92-2435

54. Boundary issues take on new meanings when you're the only psychiatrist around. Psychiatric News, Nov 17, 1995, p 6

# APPENDIX 2

## Suggested Readings

Clinicians interested in furthering their study of going to court may find the following references valuable:

Appelbaum PS, Gutheil TG: Clinical Handbook of Psychiatry and the Law. Baltimore, MD, Williams & Wilkins, 1991 (See especially Chapters 7 and 8.)

Brodsky SL: Testifying in Court: Guidelines and Maxims for the Expert Witness. Washington, DC, American Psychological Association, 1991 (An admittedly more advanced work for experts, and with some idiosyncratic views [e.g., no tie], but with many good tips.)

Charles SC, Kennedy E: Defendant: A Psychiatrist on Trial for Medical Malpractice. New York, Free Press, 1985 (Still among the best first-person accounts.)

Danner D: Medical Malpractice: A Primer for Physicians. Boston, MA, Lawyers' Cooperative, 1988 (For the latest version, write to Douglas Danner, Esq., Powers and Hall, 100 Franklin St., Boston, MA 02110.)

Greenberg SA, Shuman DW: Irreconcilable conflict between therapeutic and forensic roles. Professional Psychology: Research and Practice 28:50–57, 1997 (An excellent review of the topic, complementary to Appendix 1 in this volume.)

Group for the Advancement of Psychiatry, Committee on Psychiatry and Law: Report 131: The Mental Health Professional and the Legal System. New York, Brunner/Mazel, 1991 (See especially Sections 5, 8, 9, 12, and 13.)

Gutheil TG, Bursztajn H, Brodsky A, et al: Decision Making in Psychiatry and Law. Baltimore, MD, Williams & Wilkins, 1991 (Chapter 1 is the anatomy of a malpractice trial from beginning to end; many useful comments.)

Halleck SL: Law in the Practice of Psychiatry. New York, Plenum, 1980 (See especially Parts I and III.)

Resnick PJ: The psychiatrist in court, in Psychiatry, Vol 3. Edited by Cavenar JO. Philadelphia, PA, JB Lippincott, 1986, pp 1–10 (A short overview by one of the deans of forensic psychiatry.)

Simon RI: Clinical Psychiatry and the Law, 2nd Edition. Washington, DC, American Psychiatric Press, 1992

# Index